BrainRecovery.com

Powerful Therapy for Challenging Brain Disorders

David Perlmutter, M.D.
Board Certified Neurologist

The Perlmutter Health Center
Naples, Florida
USA

This book has been written and published to provide information and should not be used as a substitute for the recommendations of your medical doctor. Because each person and medical situation are unique, the reader is urged to review this information with a qualified health professional. You should not consider the information contained in this text to represent the practice of medicine or to replace consultation with a physician or other qualified healthcare provider.

Published by   **The Perlmutter Health Center**
                800 Goodlette Road North, Suite 270
                Naples, Fl 34102   USA
                (239) 649-7400

ISBN: 0-9635874-1-2

Printed in the United States of America
Second printing, August, 2000
Third printing, May, 2001
Fourth printing, January, 2003

Contents

Acknowledgements   v

Foreword   vii
  By Dr. Bernie Siegel

Foreword   ix
  By Dr. Jeffrey Bland

Introduction   1

1. Parkinson's Disease   11
2. Multiple Sclerosis   37
3. Amyotrophic Lateral Sclerosis   67
4. Post-Polio Syndrome   85
5. Alzheimer's Disease   99
6. Vascular Dementia   127
7. Stroke Recovery   133
8. Brain Protection and Performance Enhancement   151
9. Hyperbaric Oxygen Therapy   165

About the author   174

Glossary   175

Index   178

Acknowledgements

I would like to thank my wife Leize, not only for sharing the vision and providing the motivation to make this book become a reality, but in addition for her continuing loving support during its production,

To our children, Austin and Reisha, thank you for understanding how important it has been for me to write this book.

I am grateful to Dr. Bernie Siegel, not just for his gracious foreword, but also for his guidance and encouragement when I began this journey so many years ago.

I join an ever-increasing cadre of physicians who owe words of gratitude to Dr. Jeffrey S. Bland whose ability to distill relevant information from the vastness of scientific research and present it coherently to our eager minds truly exemplifies the meaning of the word doctor.

Finally, I wish to thank my father, Irwin Perlmutter, M.D., for providing an incredible example of compassion and joy for the healing arts. After 45 years of practicing neurosurgery, he is now creating a free clinic for indigent care in North Carolina – in his 84th year.

Dad, when you're ready to pass the torch, I hope I carry it half as well as you.

Foreword

I have just finished reading Dr. David Perlmutter's book, BrainRecovery.com – *Powerful Therapy for Challenging Brain Disorders,* and have sat in awe of both what is happening in neurology and the manner in which Dr. Perlmutter tells the story. In my education thirty years ago, I learned that brain injury was irreversible and that disorders such as Parkinson's and Alzheimer's were inherited. What I learn from both the scholarship and clinical expertise of Dr. Perlmutter in his book is that both of these concepts are wrong. The brain, to some extent, can be healed and these neurological diseases are not predetermined and unmodifiable.

What a tremendous sense of empowerment for the individual who is either at risk or who has early stage neurodegenerative disease to know that there is something that can be done.

I applaud Dr. Perlmutter for making this breakthrough information available not only to the medical community, but more importantly, to the many people who need to learn of it. It was only in the early 1990's that the concepts of brain plasticity and brain healing started to be better understood by the biomedical community. It might be another ten years before it is widely understood and in general medical practice by the average physician. Dr. Perlmutter's book gives the reader at least a ten-year head start in accessing this revolutionary information for their own health and those for whom this information can be vitally important.

Jeffrey Bland, Ph.D.
President, Institute for Functional Medicine

Foreword

I am writing this foreword not because I am a neurologist capable of evaluating the entire book's contents, but because I am someone who has chosen to have my family members and patients cared for by Doctor David Perlmutter. I deeply respect his open-mindedness and expertise as a physician. He combines the skills of a well trained traditional medical practitioner and caring physician with the wisdom of one who goes beyond the limitations of today's so called medical education and the closed–minded medicine I see practiced today.

As one who has been working for over twenty years to enlighten medical minds to treat the whole person and integrate their care, I see David as a leader in his field. He is willing to explore new therapeutic modalities - skillfully and compassionately guiding his patients through challenging medical problems. His book is an excellent resource based upon his extensive experience and expertise in areas others are often slow to accept because of their training and limited information.

On a personal level I know the struggles I have gone through to receive therapies that David now makes available to patients through his practice and consultations. He and his book are true guides for those who seek healing. The information contained needs to be available to everyone so true integrative therapy can become the normal method of treatment in the field of neurology.

Bernie Siegel, M.D.

Introduction

The end of the 1990's marked the completion of the so-called *Decade of the Brain,* a title bestowed upon this period by researchers and clinicians in the neurosciences not only to enhance awareness of the various neurodegenerative diseases, but also to encourage research into the diverse genetic, infectious, environmental, traumatic and life-style influences on their development. But despite the commendable advances in our understanding of the causes of these maladies, lack of significant progress from a therapeutic perspective may mean that we will leave the Decade of the Brain to usher in the *Century of Brain Dysfunction.*

Our understanding of the possible underlying causes of Alzheimer's disease, including genetic predisposition, educational level, electromagnetic radiation, aluminum exposure, and estrogen insufficiency, has advanced dramatically. But despite the encouraging claims in medical journal advertisements, none of the currently marketed "Alzheimer's drugs" offers any significant benefit for this devastating disease. Indeed as the highly respected *Journal of the American Medical Association* recently reported in a comprehensive review of the effectiveness of tacrine (Cognex®), one of the most aggressively marketed drugs for Alzheimer's disease, "Despite being licensed in several countries, the efficacy of tacrine in treating the symptoms of Alzheimer's disease remains controversial, and government approval for its use has been refused in several countries."[1]

These are sobering comments from a journal looked upon as the sounding board of American medicine, especially in light of the fact that there are an estimated 4.5 million Alzheimer's patients in the United States today, and caring for these individuals costs the nation more than $60 billion annually. But these statistics pale when confronting projections for the next 30 years. Alzheimer's, being primarily a disease of the aged, will have an ever-increasing impact on our

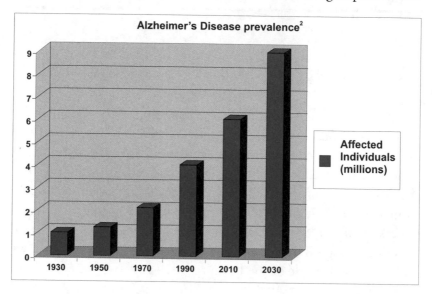

Alzheimer's Disease prevalence[2]

society as the elderly represent the most rapidly growing segment of our population. As seen above, by 2030 we can anticipate over 9 million Alzheimer's patients in this country with close to *half* the population over 85 years carrying the diagnosis.[2]

The situation is much the same with other degenerative diseases of the nervous system. Between the years 1955-1986, the mortality from Parkinson's disease in the U.S. rose a staggering 411% while deaths from amyotrophic lateral sclerosis (ALS or Lou Gehrig's disease) increased an astounding 328% in the 9-year period from 1977 to 1986.[3]

But is the rapid increase of these diseases simply a reflection of the fact that we are now living longer and not succumbing to other processes? Or are there other influential factors in our society which have a bearing on these degenerative conditions? An attempt to answer this question appeared in a 1993 editorial in the Journal *The Lancet* in which the author stated, "Modern civilization is not the cause of our chronic diseases, it merely unveiled what our genes had lurking in store for us for centuries, if not millennia, as we now live long enough to see these genes massively expressing themselves."[4]

This idea, that our health is entirely determined by our genes, suggests that our fate with respect to neurodegenerative conditions is predetermined at the time of our conception. Environmental, nutritional and emotional aspects of our lives have little influence in this perspective. Progression of disease is inherent in this plan, allowing perhaps only a role for treating *symptoms* – paying attention only to the smoke and not the underlying fire.

But in the past several years, the vigorous explorations of the fundamental biochemical events involved in the progressive deterioration of the nervous system characteristic of the neurodegenerative diseases have revealed that these conditions do not simply represent a linear predetermined progression. The unbending rules of genetic determinism have been replaced by the paradigm of *genetic predisposition* – a

By 2030 we can anticipate over 9 million Alzheimer's patients in this country.

concept that recognizes inherited risk as being one of many factors that influences an individual's ability to resist the entropic nature of the tenuous forces maintaining nervous system integrity.

The molecular mechanism underlying nervous system decay characteristic of these disorders shares a final common pathway with the process of aging in everything living. The key players mediating this degeneration belong to a group of chemicals commonly known as *free radicals*.

Despite the negativity associated with these molecules in popular health texts, free radicals mediate processes central to the perpetuation of life itself. In humans, free radicals direct the formation of our various body parts, initiate and modulate immune activity, execute invading bacteria, and destroy cancer cells.

Free radicals are generated during the normal processes of cellular metabolism and are produced in increased amounts when physiologic systems are stressed. Stressors associated with increased free radical production may be intrinsic, as occurs for example when emotion induces the production of "stress hormones," or when blood supply is compromised. Extrinsic influences known to stimulate free radical production include such diverse events as infection, trauma, exposure to toxins, and irradiation.

It is when the controlling mechanisms normally limiting the life span or activity of free radicals become inadequate that the destructive nature of these short-lived molecules becomes manifest. This occurs when excessive free radicals overwhelm the body's protective antioxidant chemicals, or antioxidant insufficiency prevents adequate protection from even the normal level of free radical production.

Within each living cell in the human body there exist microscopic particles whose sole purpose is energy production. These inclusions, the *mitochondria,* are responsible for utilizing fuel to provide power for all of the cell's various activities. But despite their critical role in maintaining the life of the cell, mitochondria are unusually susceptible to being damaged by free radicals. When damaged, mitochondrial energy production suffers, rendering the entire cell, including the mitochondria, even more susceptible to free radical damage. And to make matters worse, this entire process becomes self-perpetuating as damaged mitochondria produce excessive amounts of free radicals as depicted below.

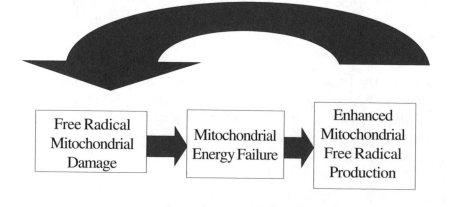

| Free Radical Mitochondrial Damage | → | Mitochondrial Energy Failure | → | Enhanced Mitochondrial Free Radical Production |

What emerges is a vicious cycle culminating in cell death which may be initiated by various factors. Alzheimer's disease is characterized by an inherent defect in mitochondrial energy production, an inflammatory response to one or more brain proteins, increased amounts of brain iron, and ineffective antioxidant activity. All of these factors contribute to a hostile environment for delicate brain neurons by enhancing free radical damage.

In Parkinson's disease the theme is much the same with a primary flaw in mitochondrial energy production and increased free radical enhancing brain iron. Inflammation is less of a factor, but unique to this disease are defects in the ability of the liver to detoxify various environmental toxins. These flaws allow accumulation of diverse chemical agents which directly compromise mitochondrial function and enhance the destructive potential of free radicals. The failure of perhaps the most critical of nervous system antioxidants, *glutathione*, is now accepted as a pivotal player in the brain destruction characteristic of Parkinson's disease. This is why therapy designed to increase glutathione activity plays a major role in the BrainRecovery.com protocol for Parkinson's disease.

Excessive free radical activity is a hallmark of multiple sclerosis as a consequence of inflammation induced by an uninhibited immune reaction directed at *myelin*, the fragile protective insulation surrounding brain neurons. The damaging effects of this misdirected immune response are compounded by antioxidant inadequacies characteristic of this disease as well.

The fundamentals of ALS remain somewhat more obscure. Increased incidence in individuals with a history of pesticide exposure suggests abnormalities of liver detoxification as is seen in Parkinson's disease. Although the focus of intensive research during the 1980's, the idea that ALS may represent a misdirected immune reaction is now less popular, while excessive free radical production from damaged mitochondria is now well accepted.[5]

Even more elusive is the nature of the underlying pathology in post-polio syndrome. In this disease, patients who had experienced polio at an earlier time in their lives, face a progressive disease beginning decades after the original event. Clearly the destruction of nerve cells is mediated by free radicals, but what triggers the recurrence of this activity remains unknown.

As diverse as the symptoms of these various conditions may appear, it should now seem clear that they share two fundamental elements mediating cellular degeneration:

- Defective antioxidant protection
- Reduced mitochondrial energy production

Thus, therapeutic strategies targeting these fundamental elements are applicable to all the neurodegenerative conditions. This approach has yielded remarkable results. The simple fat-soluble antioxidant vitamin E has been reported in *The New England Journal of Medicine* to be more effective in Alzheimer's disease than *any* pharmaceutical agent available.[6]

Even more powerful antioxidants are now available, promising to take brain protection to a much higher level. Perhaps

Enhancing the energy producing ability of mitochondria is the key to revitalizing brain tissue.

the most exciting of this new breed of antioxidants is *alpha lipoic acid*. Having the unique attributes of being rapidly absorbed from the gut, readily crossing the blood-brain barrier, and having powerful free radical scavenging activity, alpha lipoic acid will likely revolutionize the treatment of all the neurodegenerative diseases. In addition to its own antioxidant activity, alpha lipoic acid also facilitates the regeneration of all the other major brain antioxidants including vitamins C and E, and glutathione. It is no wonder that this nutrient derived antioxidant is the subject of intensive scientific evaluation.

While the critical antioxidant glutathione cannot be effectively administered orally, its production can be dramatically enhanced by providing N-acetyl-cysteine (NAC), a nutritional supplement soon to share the spotlight with lipoic acid.

Manipulation of dietary fatty acids provides a potent technique to reduce the free radical generation associated with the inflammation in multiple sclerosis. The role of inflammation has now been secured as one of the major players responsible for free radical generation in Alzheimer's disease as well, bringing dietary manipulation to the forefront as a therapeutic modality in this ever increasing illness.

Enhancing the energy producing ability of mitochondria is the key to revitalizing brain tissue. A host of potent substances including *phosphatidylserine, acetyl-L-carnitine, Ginkgo biloba, coenzyme Q10,* and *NADH,* have each been extensively studied, with reports substantiating their profound effectiveness appearing in our most highly regarded scientific journals.

In addition to the neurodegenerative diseases, this book reveals powerful therapies for stroke, cerebral palsy, and brain trauma – all considered nonprogressive disorders. While ongoing free radical damage is less an issue in these conditions, defective mitochondrial energy production becomes the key factor maintaining disability after injury.

Whether an area of the brain is damaged by trauma, compromised blood supply (stroke), or prenatal injury (cerebral palsy), the gradient between healthy, normally functioning brain tissue and areas of completely dysfunctional neurons is indistinct. It is in the intermediate zones between the healthy and severely damaged tissue where a population of cells exists that although damaged, are still able to be brought back online with appropriate therapy. These neurons have been termed "idling neurons" – an appropriate title for cells functional but not functioning. Enhancing mitochondrial energy production is the key to reestablishing function in these cells. Exciting strategies are now available to accomplish this task, ultimately leading to clinical improvement.

Among the most potent techniques now available to enhance the activity of marginally functioning neurons is *hyperbaric oxygen therapy* (HBOT). This therapy involves exposing patients to life-giving oxygen under conditions of increased atmospheric pressure. While HBOT has been recognized and utilized for several decades as a potent therapy for stroke recovery, multiple sclerosis, head injury and cerebral palsy across Europe and Asia, the United States, for the most part, has failed to embrace its usefulness. No doubt the lack of recognition of the therapeutic potential of hyperbaric oxygen, like the many potent nutritional supplements mentioned above, stems from the inability of any one company to obtain an exclusive patent on its use or distribution. This precludes these approaches from being the focus of major advertising dollars – the real key to being recognized by most healthcare practitioners.

This likely explains why most readers of this book are unaware that *vinpocetine,* a simple extract of the periwinkle plant, is revolutionizing therapy for stroke recovery across Europe and Japan. By augmenting brain blood flow to areas of marginal function, vinpocetine enhances the provision of oxygen and nutrients to neurons anxious to

A simple extract of the periwinkle plant, is revolutionizing therapy for stroke recovery across Europe and Japan.

resume their previous level of activity. The clinical studies substantiating its effectiveness are extensive, and are reviewed in this text.

BrainRecovery.com should not be looked upon as providing "alternative therapy." This designation connotes a decision making process where one approach is used to the exclusion of others. Rather, this information should be used to *complement* many of the vast array of therapies offered by conventional medicine.

Reluctance on the part of conventional practitioners to embrace or even consider complementary approaches is typically (and frequently erroneously) justified by statements indicating a lack of "peer reviewed studies" or "scientific evidence." The therapeutic techniques described in this text are supported by literature citations from the most respected, peer reviewed scientific and medical publications on the planet.

As we are now firmly entrenched in the "information age," the knowledge we so desperately need to maintain health and meet the challenges of disease is finally within our grasp. Our dependence upon a system where standard of care is dictated by pharmaceutical advertising is giving way to a new standard of care – one that recognizes the utility of a wide spectrum of well-studied, scientifically validated interventions not solely disseminated by the prescription pad.

It has been said that knowledge is power, but clearly in this context, *knowledge is health.*

References

[1] Qizilbash, N., Whitehead, A., Higgins, J., et al., Cholinesterase Inhibition for Alzheimer's Disease – A Meta-analysis of the Tacrine Trials. JAMA 280L1777-1782,1998

[2] Cumings J.L., Current Perspectives in Alzheimer's disease. Neurology 51 (suppl. 1): S1,1998

[3] Riggs, Jack E., The Aging Population – Implications for the Burden of Neurologic Disease. In Riggs, J.(ed.) *Neurologic Clinics*, Philadelphia, W.B. Saunders p.556, 1998

[4] Editorial: Rise and Fall of Diseases. Lancet,341:151-52, 1993

[5] Rothstein, J.D., Martin, L.J., Kuncl, R.W. Decreased glutamate transport by the brain and spinal cord in amyotrophic lateral sclerosis. N Eng J Med 236:1464-68, 1992

[6] Sano, M., Ernesto, C., Thomas, R.G., et al., A controlled trial of selegeline, alpha-tocopherol, or both as treatment for Alzheimer's disease. N Engl J Med 336:1216-22, 1997

CHAPTER ONE

Parkinson's Disease

It has been estimated that in the United States alone more than 1 million people have Parkinson's disease, with more than 50,000 new cases being diagnosed each year. That translates to a prevalence of about 1-2 cases per 1000 individuals in the general population. This prevalence increases dramatically when looking at the over 55 population, approaching 1 in 100. The average age of onset is about 60 years, but it may be diagnosed as early as the mid 30's.[1] Perhaps because of some brain protective effects of female hormones, men are slightly more at risk than women.

Symptoms of Parkinson's disease vary from patient to patient but typically include tremor, rigidity, slowness of movement, and disturbances of posture. The tremor of the Parkinsonian patient is somewhat characteristic in that unlike other forms of tremor, it is worse at rest and may improve substantially when the affected limb is used. It is worse with stress and typically begins on one side, usually affecting the hand. Thereafter, the opposite hand may become involved as well as other parts of the body including the legs, facial muscles and even the tongue.

The rigidity in Parkinson's may involve any of the major limbs. Typically there is increased tone throughout the range of motion of the involved joint.

Slowness of movement, technically known as *bradykinesia*, is another hallmark of the disease and can be one of the most incapacitating symptoms. Patients report difficulty in initiating movements and may have great difficulty in arising from a chair or starting to walk when standing. They may describe a sensation of feeling like they are wearing "cement boots," or that their feet are "magnetic." Facial expressions are reduced, and it may be difficult to begin speaking. The handwriting may become smaller and patients may find it difficult to turn over in bed.

As the disease progresses, the posture becomes affected with increased forward flexion at the waist and a tendency to stand and walk in a stooped position. As Dr. James Parkinson described in his original 1817 monograph:

"After a few more months the patient is found to be less strict in preserving the upright posture: this being most observable whilst walking, but sometimes whilst sitting or standing. Sometime after the appearance of this symptom, and during its slow increase, one of the legs is discovered slightly to tremble, and is also found to suffer fatigue sooner than the leg of the other side: and in a few months this limb becomes agitated by similar tremblings, and suffers a similar loss of power." [2]

The Glutathione Miracle

It has long been recognized that a fundamental abnormality in Parkinson's disease patients is the failure of a specific part of the brain, the *substantia nigra*, to produce an important brain chemical, the neurotransmitter *dopamine*. Focusing on this specific chemical flaw, the pharmaceutical industry has developed a wide array of medications to provide symptomatic relief.

In 1959 the first true therapeutic approach to treating the symptoms of Parkinson's disease *L-dopa therapy may actually increase free radical production.* was proposed attempting to replace dopamine. This is the basis for the use of the dopamine derivative L-dopa (Sinemet®) in the treatment of Parkinson's disease symptoms.[3] Indeed, even today L-dopa therapy remains the mainstay of treatment. Unfortunately, while L-dopa therapy may help to temporarily reduce the symptoms of Parkinson's disease, many scientific reports are now appearing in medical journals warning that L-dopa therapy may actually increase free radical production and thus speed up the progression of the illness, causing patients to worsen more quickly.[4]

With so much emphasis placed on L-dopa therapy, it is important to recognize that another vital brain chemical is also profoundly deficient in Parkinson's disease. This chemical, glutathione, is substantially reduced, virtually across the board, in Parkinson's patients. And yet, this deficiency seems to receive precious little attention.[5]

Glutathione is a critically important brain chemical. It is clearly one of the most important brain antioxidants. That is, glutathione helps to preserve brain tissue by preventing damage from free radicals - destructive chemicals formed by the normal processes of metabolism, toxic elements in the environment, and as a normal response of the body to challenges by infectious agents or other stresses. In addition to quenching dangerous free radicals, glutathione also acts to recycle vitamin C and vitamin E, which, because of their antioxidant activity, also reduce free radicals in the brain.

"All patients improved significantly after glutathione therapy, with a 42% decline in disability."

So, with the understanding that glutathione is important for brain protection, and that this protection may be lacking in the brains of Parkinson's patients because of their glutathione deficiency, wouldn't it make sense to give glutathione to Parkinson's patients experimentally and observe their outcome? That's exactly what was done in a landmark study from the *Department of Neurology, University of Sassari, Italy*. In this research protocol, Parkinson's patients received intravenous glutathione twice daily for 30 days. The subjects were then evaluated at one month intervals for up to six months. The published results indicated "all patients improved significantly after glutathione therapy, with a 42% decline in disability. Once glutathione was stopped, the therapeutic effect lasted 2-4 months." Further, the researchers indicated "...glutathione has symptomatic efficacy and possibly retards the progression of the disease." [6]

It is unclear exactly why this study has remained almost completely unrecognized. In the United States, the use of L-dopa, or other drugs designed to mimic it, remains the standard of care. And yet, this Italian study demonstrated that giving glutathione, a substance naturally occurring in the brain, provided Parkinson's patients substantial benefit.

Glutathione as such, cannot be patented. So it cannot be owned exclusively by any particular pharmaceutical company and therefore won't find its way to the highly influential advertising sections of the medical journals. And yet, quite simply we know that the brains of Parkinson's patients are profoundly deficient in this important chemical, with clinical research supporting its incredible effectiveness.

We began administering intravenous glutathione in late 1998. The effectiveness of this brain antioxidant in Parkinson's disease is nothing short of miraculous. Certainly, its administration is more complicated than simply "taking a pill," but on the other hand, there are essentially no reported side effects. In addition, while our Parkinson's patients are now realizing profound improvements with respect to reduction of rigidity, increased mobility, improved ability to speak, less depression, and decreased tremor, glutathione has the added benefit of protecting the brain from free radical damage, thus *slowing* the progression of the underlying illness. This contrasts so vividly with the simplistic approach of only treating symptoms while potentially worsening the underlying disease.

Following even a single dosage of intravenous glutathione, many of the symptoms of Parkinson's disease are rapidly improved, often, in as little as 15 minutes. Injections are typically repeated from 3 times a week to as often as daily.

Here is an example of a typical response to glutathione therapy in a patient with moderately advanced Parkinson's disease:

Dear Dr. Perlmutter:

This letter is to advise you of the progress of my husband's response to the glutathione therapy started two weeks ago.

As you know (HS), now 72 years old, had been diagnosed with Parkinson's disease five years ago, starting with a tremor in his right hand. The disease progressed rapidly, impairing his walking ability, balance, and reducing his voice volume and clarity. Most recently, his inability to walk had made it necessary for him to use a wheelchair when leaving the house. At home, he has used a walker for the past two years.

His prescribed medications have included Sinemet®, Mirapex®, and Tasmar® over the past years, the effects of which have diminished.

Almost immediately after your first treatment of glutathione IV two weeks ago, there was a marked improvement in his facial expression, his voice volume, and ability to walk and turn. He started with 400 mg., 3 times a week. The effective period of time after injection has increased from one hour to almost the whole day. When we visited your office last he received 600 mg., and his ability to walk almost normally lasted the full day and part of the next.

He also reports that he has a general feeling of wellbeing after each treatment. And he is now taking 400 units of glutathione IV once a day, together with the supplements you have prescribed.

We are thrilled to report that he has not used the wheelchair for the past two days and is able to take full strides with his arm linked in mine. His facial expression is animated and his voice volume has increased.

In addition, we have cut back on his intake of Sinemet® and stopped the Tasmar®. In the past, without the Sinemet®, he had been unable to walk – his legs practically frozen. With the glutathione therapy, he can walk with a reduced intake of Sinemet®.

We feel our prayers have been answered—that there is something positive that can be done to fight and arrest this dreadful disease now. We cannot thank you enough for the hope you have given us and we will keep you informed as to his progress until the next office visit.

Most consider Parkinson's disease to be an affliction only of the elderly. But we are now seeing patients in their 50's, 40's, and even 30's, with regularity. Here is a report from a 57-year-old plastic surgeon and former marathon runner:

Dear David:

This is a follow up since my visit with you in April of 1999. As you will recall, my symptoms were those of micrographia (small handwriting), drooling, exhaustion, tremor, inanimate facies, poor voice projection and modulation, and depression. Your diagnosis was that of Parkinson's disease. I was started on glutathione 400 mg, three times a week, and I was instructed to take vitamins D, E, and B12 in addition to my rather extensive vitamin and herbal supplementation program.

I received my first dose of glutathione in your office that day and within two hours I felt like a new person. I was more animate and expressive almost immediately. Over the next few weeks, my voice became stronger, I felt less tired and my tremor almost disappeared. More slowly, my writing has improved; it's not perfect (never was) but at least with effort and slowing down, I can write legibly now. I still tend to drool some but even that is much improved. My energy is not totally back to normal but I am working a full schedule as a plastic surgeon with a very busy practice. My depression is gone and I have my sense of humor back.

When I was originally diagnosed at Duke, I was given a prescription for Sinemet® and advised to get my affairs in order. Your approach has kept me off this medication, almost restored me to normal, and more importantly, has given me hope that we may slow the progression of my disease if not halt it altogether.

I want you to know how very much I appreciate your care, your caring, and your pioneering efforts.

Thank you.

There are several factors that explain why glutathione is so beneficial in Parkinson's disease. First, glutathione has the unique ability to make certain areas of the brain more sensitive to dopamine, so that even though dopamine is decreased, it nevertheless becomes more effective.[7] The concept of enhancing cellular receptor sensitivity has become quite familiar in medicine today. In diabetes for example, before actually administering insulin, physicians often begin therapy by prescribing the drug *metformin,* which acts by enhancing the sensitivity of cells to whatever insulin is still being produced.

In addition, as mentioned above, glutathione has profound antioxidant activity – protecting the brain from free radical damage. But an even more intriguing benefit of glutathione lies not in the brain but in an area of the body far beyond the scope of typical neurology.

The Liver Connection

Glutathione is one of the most important components of the liver's detoxification system. It has long been recognized that most Parkinson's patients manifest flaws in their ability to detoxify various chemicals to which they are exposed. This is the obvious explanation as to why Parkinson's disease is so much more prevalent in individuals with *Parkinson's patients manifest flaws in their ability to detoxify various chemicals to which they are exposed.* a history of occupational exposure to agricultural pesticides or various other toxic chemicals.[8] While not every person exposed to pesticides or other toxins develops Parkinson's disease, those unfortunate few who harbor an inherited flaw in their detoxification pathways are at far greater risk to the brain damaging effects of a wide variety of toxins as we described in 1997.[9]

Giving glutathione is one of the most effective techniques for enhancing liver and brain detoxification. The nutritional supplement N-acetyl-cysteine, (often abbreviated NAC), enhances the body's production of glutathione and thus aids the detoxification process. Other nutritional supplements which enhance glutathione and thus aid in detoxification include vitamins E and C, alpha lipoic acid, and the herb *silymarin.*

MediClear® a nutritional supplement designed by *Thorne Research, Inc,* to enhance hepatic and bowel detoxification, and for systemic inflammatory control and allergy relief. *MediClear®* can also be used to treat increased gut permeability, dysbiosis, and gastrointestinal inflammation.

Enhancing liver detoxification can have a dramatic effect on the manifestations of Parkinson's disease as exemplified by the following case history:

> *Report of a Case*: B.K. is a 40-year-old male who, in 1989 at the age of 34, began experiencing a tremor of the right hand. This was associated with micrographia (small handwriting) and the subsequent development of a right leg tremor. Over the next several years he developed slowness of movement, a reduction of facial expression, and a prominent loss of arm swinging when walking. He was placed on a sustained release preparation of L-dopa (Sinemet CR®) which produced a definite improvement of his symptoms.
>
> When evaluated on 10/10/95, his medications included sustained release L-dopa (Sinemet CR® 25/100) three times each day, standard release L-dopa (Sinemet 25/100) twice each day, selegiline (Eldepryl®) 5 mg twice each day, and bromocriptine (Parlodel®) 5 mg twice a day. As with many of our patients, a videotape recording was made to document his clinical status.
>
> His past medical history revealed that he had lived directly adjacent to a large commercial pesticide-using farm for the first twelve years of his life, and he recalled how he and his friends would follow the pesticide spraying tractors through the corn fields for fun.

On 02/06/96, the patient began a two-week nutritional program designed to improve liver detoxification. After the initial two weeks the patient reported, "My medications are working better and I have much less rigidity and tremor." These findings were confirmed on the physical examination. Videotape recording was made prior to and subsequent to the treatment protocol, and a significant improvement was also noted in fluidity of movement, facial expression, and arm movement with walking. Perhaps even more impressive was the fact that these improvements persisted, even after the medications were markedly reduced.

At follow up examination *three years* after the initial detoxification he demonstrated continued improvement of clinical symptoms compared to his initial videotaped exam, and he remains on a reduced schedule of medications.

Evaluating an individual's detoxification status is easily accomplished using a very simple test, the *Hepatic Detoxification Profile* available from the *Great Smokies Diagnostic Laboratory* in Asheville, North Carolina (see below). The test involves the oral administration of several over-the-counter challenge substances. Subsequently, saliva, urine and blood are collected and analyzed to determine how these substances are metabolized. The results provide an extremely comprehensive picture of the various liver detoxification pathways, allowing the treating physician to design a specific interventional program to improve liver function.

Finally, keep in mind that certain drugs can reduce liver detoxification function. Acetaminophen, a drug commonly used for pain and fever, can actually reduce liver glutathione and should therefore be avoided.[10] It is found in a large number of over-the-counter and prescription medications, so pay close attention to labels.

Cellular Activation

During the 1990's, the so-called *"Decade of the Brain,"* scientists learned that the fundamental flaw not allowing certain brain cells to produce dopamine in the Parkinson's patient is a deficiency in the actual *energetics* of these cells. It is as if these cells, while still alive, are simply unable to produce the energy needed for normal activity. Incredibly, the most widely prescribed medication for Parkinson's disease, L-dopa (Sinemet®), has been shown to actually lead to further compromise of the brains ability to produce energy.[11] This further reduces the production of dopamine, leading to worsening of the disease.

With a formal understanding of the biochemistry of energy production, researchers have explored a variety of interventions designed to "jump start" these lethargic cells, often with dramatic results. And best of all, most of the research has involved non-pharmacological products. The most promising of these cellular activators are NADH , CoQ10, and phosphatidylserine.

NADH (Nicotinamide Adenine Dinucleotide)

NADH is an enzyme which has a pivotal role in energy production in all living cells, and particularly in brain cells. The amount of energy a cell can produce is directly related to NADH availability. Since Parkinson's disease represents a failure of cellular energy production, it's reasonable that researchers would take a look at NADH as a potential therapeutic agent.

Pioneering work published by Dr. Jörg Birkmayer in 1993 revealed just how potent NADH can be as part of a comprehensive program for the Parkinson's patient. Of 885 patients who received NADH in his study, an astounding 80% showed "moderate to excellent improvements in their disability."[12] This shouldn't come as a surprise given NADH's profound effectiveness in other neurological disorders including Alzheimer's disease (see chapter five).

Coenzyme Q10 (CoQ10)

The other important player in energy production is CoQ10. Like NADH, CoQ10 is also present in all living cells where it too plays a critical role in cellular energy production. Energy deficiencies in specific parts of the brain can produce inadequate production of important brain chemicals. And, according to Dr. M. Flint Beal at the *Massachusetts General Hospital*, Parkinson's patients demonstrate a profound deficiency of coenzyme Q10 which may explain why their brains produce an inadequate supply of dopamine. Interestingly, Dr. Beal's research revealed that not only was coenzyme Q10 deficient in Parkinson's patients, but in their spouses as well - although to a lesser extent (see figure1.1).[13] This unexpected finding lends further support to the concept that Parkinson's disease may in

Parkinson's patients demonstrate a profound deficiency of coenzyme Q10

some way be related to some extrinsic environmental factor.

The encouraging news from Dr. Beal's research is that orally administered CoQ10 is readily absorbed, well tolerated, and measurably increases cellular energy production.[14] These qualities, coupled with its profound antioxidant properties, likely explain why the therapeutic potential of CoQ10 in Parkinson's disease is now the subject of intensive research at major medical institutions all across the country.

Finally, recognizing the importance of coenzyme Q10 makes it critical to identify any factors which may lower its availability. Unfortunately, two of the most commonly prescribed cholesterol lowering drugs, pravastatin (Pravachol®) and lovastatin (Mevacor®), dramatically lower serum coenzyme Q10 levels.[15]

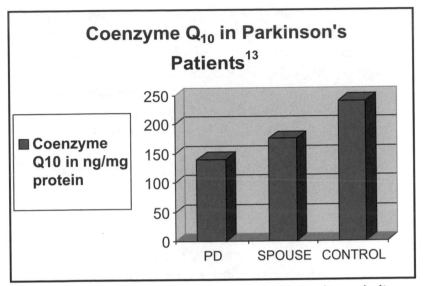

Coenzyme Q_{10} in Parkinson's Patients[13]

Figure 1.1. Relative levels of coenzyme Q10 in Parkinson's disease (PD) patients, their spouses, and controls.

Phosphatidylserine

Phosphatidylserine is one of the key components of *neuronal membranes* - the site where brain cells both receive and transmit chemical messages. Enhancing chemical transmission is of obvious importance in Parkinson's disease, an illness in which the fundamental abnormality is a flaw in the ability of neurons to communicate chemically because of a deficiency of dopamine. Even in the face of this deficiency, increasing phosphatidylserine may enhance the effectiveness of what little dopamine remains – helping to preserve brain function.

The energy producing mitochondria also rely upon a healthy membrane to carry out the function of energy production. Like the cellular membrane, the mitochondrial membrane requires adequate phosphatidylserine to maintain normal function.

It has been estimated that as many as 30% of Parkinson's disease patients suffer from a progressive decline not only in motor function but in cognitive ability as well. At times the dementia associated with the disease is more debilitating than the common problems of tremor, rigidity and balance disorders. This further supports the inclusion of phosphatidylserine in treating Parkinson's disease since research supports its profound therapeutic potential in dementia. This was confirmed in a 1991 article in the journal *Neurology* in which researchers from *Stanford University* demonstrated a marked improvement on performance tests related to memory and learning in a group of 149 memory impaired patients treated with phosphatidylserine for 12 weeks.[16]

Antioxidant Protection

As in other neurodegenerative diseases, antioxidants have an important role in protecting the brain in Parkinson's disease – a disease characterized by excessive free radical production coupled with deficient antioxidant defenses. This is not a new concept. The research exploring both the role of free radicals and the protective effects of antioxidants in diseases like Parkinson's goes back at least 2 decades. In a 1988 report entitled *"Case-control study of early life dietary factors in Parkinson's disease"* published in *Archives of Neurology*, researchers discovered that simple dietary sources of vitamin E *profoundly* reduced the risk of Parkinson's disease. Compared to controls, those who consumed diets rich in nuts had a risk of Parkinson's disease only 39% of controls. Consumers of seed based salad dressings had a risk only 30% of normal, while consumption of plums was associated with a risk reduced to an incredible 24% of the average population.[17]

Unfortunately, vitamin and nutritional information is not typically conveyed on the prescription pad - the ultimate coin of medical commerce.

Retrospective epidemiological studies like these have prompted research to determine if administering antioxidants could slow the progression of disease in those already diagnosed. Dr. Stanley Fahn, one of the country's most highly respected neurologists and chairman of the *Department of Neurology* at *Columbia University College of Physicians and Surgeons*, evaluated the effectiveness of vitamins E and C in a large group of Parkinson's patients over several years. At the beginning of the study, none of the patients was debilitated enough to need the standard Parkinson's drug, L-dopa (Sinemet®). The time until patients required L-dopa therapy was extended an incredible 2.2 years in those taking these simple nonprescription vitamins.[18]

These results clearly indicate the power of antioxidants to slow the progression of Parkinson's disease. Isn't this information that should be provided to all Parkinson's patients and their families? Unfortunately, vitamin and nutritional information is not typically conveyed on the prescription pad - the ultimate coin of medical commerce.

Below is a descriptive list of powerful brain antioxidants, key players in the **BrainRecovery.com** protocol for Parkinson's disease.

Alpha Lipoic Acid

The subject of intensive study in the neurodegenerative diseases, alpha lipoic acid not only serves as an extremely powerful antioxidant in and of itself, but in addition, it regenerates vitamins C and E as well as glutathione. But unlike glutathione, which isn't useful when given orally, alpha lipoic acid is readily absorbed from the gut and has the unique ability to cross the blood-brain barrier and enter the central nervous system.

Yet another quality of alpha lipoic acid is its ability to serve as a metal chelator. That means it can bind to a variety of potentially toxic metals in the body, including cadmium and free iron, and enhance their excretion. This is an important function since these metals may increase the formation of damaging free radicals and research demonstrates substantially increased concentrations of iron in the brains of Parkinson's patients.[19]

Vitamin E

Since cell membranes and the brain in general contain large amounts of fat, vitamin E, a "fat-soluble" vitamin is particularly important in protecting the nervous system. This important brain antioxidant remains the focus of worldwide scientific evaluation for its therapeutic potential in Parkinson's disease, Alzheimer's disease and various other neurodegenerative conditions. Since Dr. Fahn's original publication in 1989, countless other researchers have confirmed the antioxidant power of this inexpensive nutritional supplement.

When buying vitamin E, always read the label carefully to ensure you are getting *d-alpha tocopherol,* not *dl-alpha tocopherol,* since the latter is synthetic and far less biologically active. Also, always refrigerate vitamin E and all other oil-based nutritional supplements to preserve their potency.

N-acetyl-cysteine (NAC)

The critical role of glutathione in the development and progression of Parkinson's disease cannot be overemphasized. While glutathione cannot be administered orally since it is readily digested to its constituent amino acids, the good news is that the nutritional supplement N-acetyl-cysteine directly encourages brain glutathione production. This activity is enhanced in the presence of adequate vitamin C and vitamin E. In addition, NAC *Viagra® works by enhancing nitric oxide production.* is itself a potent antioxidant and has been shown to specifically reduce the formation of the free radical *nitric oxide,* which has been implicated as having a causative role in Parkinson's disease, Alzheimer's disease, and several other neurodegenerative disorders.[20] Consideration of the brain damaging effects of nitric oxide is particularly timely in view of the popularity of the drug *Viagra®* which works by enhancing nitric oxide production.

Acetyl-L-carnitine

Like coenzyme Q10 and NADH, acetyl-L-carnitine enhances energy production in damaged neurons. But in addition, it is one of the most important and specific antioxidants in the BrainRecovery.com protocol for Parkinson's disease. In a fascinating study reported in 1995, researchers demonstrated the ability of acetyl-L-carnitine to completely prevent parkinsonism in laboratory animals. When laboratory animals are exposed to the brain toxin MPTP, they immediately develop full-blown parkinsonism as a consequence of enhanced production of destructive free radicals specifically in the brain area that produces dopamine. Pre-treating the animals with acetyl-L-carnitine prior to MPTP exposure offered complete protection – none of the animals developed parkinsonism. This study affirmed the potency of acetyl-L-carnitine as an antioxidant specifically useful in Parkinson's disease.[21]

Vitamin D

Although widely recognized for its role in maintaining healthy bones, vitamin D has recently become the subject of scientific interest since it too has been found to be an important antioxidant, possibly even more potent than vitamin E. In a recent (1997) study reported in the journal *Neurology*, Japanese researchers found surprisingly low levels of vitamin D in the blood of the 71 Parkinson's patients they evaluated. Not recognizing the important antioxidant, and therefore brain-protecting activity of vitamin D, these researchers simply concluded that because of their low vitamin D levels, Parkinson's disease patients are at higher risk for osteoporosis.[22, 23]

Ginkgo biloba

While widely known for its effectiveness in Alzheimer's disease, Ginkgo biloba must be included in this protocol as it too has profound brain antioxidant activity. Like acetyl-L-carnitine, Ginkgo biloba can also protect laboratory animals against the Parkinson's producing effect of the neurotoxin MPTP.[24] While humans are not typically exposed to this toxin, the idea that Parkinson's disease may be related to some other agent(s) is obviously supported by the profound increased incidence of the disease in those exposed to herbicides and other chemical agents as described above. Further, since dementia frequently complicates Parkinson's disease, inclusion of Ginkgo in the Parkinson's program makes sense, as this herb has been shown in extensive worldwide studies to enhance and preserve cognitive performance.

Vitamin C

Rounding out the list of antioxidants for Parkinson's disease is vitamin C. Having proven itself to be effective in slowing the progression of this disease in Dr. Fahn's original research, vitamin C, like vitamin E, is the focus of extensive research not only in Parkinson's disease, but in other progressive diseases of the nervous system as well. Its specific utility in Parkinson's disease was *Vitamin C helped preserve the energy producing capacity of the mitochondria.* emphasized in a study also performed by Dr. Fahn and colleagues in which it was found that vitamin C helped preserve the energy producing capacity of the mitochondria – an abnormality actually made worse by the administration of L-dopa, the most widely prescribed drug for Parkinson's disease in the country.[25]

BrainRecovery.com
Parkinson's Protocol

Intravenous Glutathione

Our protocol for using glutathione is relatively simple. Glutathione is inexpensive and easily obtained (see below). We use liquid glutathione, not reconstituted powder. It should be administered, at least initially, by a qualified healthcare practitioner as follows:

1. Dilute the appropriate dosage of glutathione liquid in 10 cc of sterile normal saline. Usually vials contain 200mg, but read the label.
2. This solution is then injected through a 21-gauge butterfly catheter intravenously over a 15 to 20 minute period of time.
3. Alternatively, many patients choose to have intravenous access ports inserted. This allows frequent glutathione administration without repeated needle sticks.
4. Treatment begins at 600mg glutathione 3 times a week and may be increased to daily injections of up to 800mg depending on results. Alternatively, a schedule of 1400mg glutathione 3 times a week may be utilized.

A complete instructional video for glutathione administration is available by calling *i*Nutritionals, at: (800) 530-1982, or may be ordered by visiting **www.BrainRecovery.com**

Injectable glutathione is available from:

> Wellness Health and Pharmaceuticals
> 2800 South 18th Street
> Birmingham, Alabama 35209
> Tel. (800) 227-2627
> Fax. (800) 369-0302

Note: It should be noted that in the fall of 2002 the Food and Drug Administration (FDA) approved research for our protocol for intravenous administration of glutathione for the treatment of Parkinson's Disease at the University of South Florida

Their web site can be accessed by visiting:
www.BrainRecovery.com

Cellular energizers

	daily dose
Coenzyme Q10	120 mg
NADH	5 mg (twice)
Phosphatidylserine	100 mg

Antioxidants

Vitamin E	1200 IU
Vitamin C	800 mg
Alpha lipoic acid	80 mg
Vitamin D	400 IU
N-acetyl-cysteine	400 mg
Acetyl-L-carnitine	400 mg
Ginkgo biloba	60 mg

Or, if using the Brain Sustain™ supplement:

Glutathione by injection, and NADH as above, and :

Brain Sustain™	2 scoops daily
Vitamin E	800 IU daily
Coenzyme Q10	60 mg daily

Note :

In Parkinson's patients less than 65 years of age check liver
detoxification by performing a:

Hepatic Detoxification Profile
available from:
Great Smokies Diagnostic Laboratory
63 Zillicoa Street
Asheville, N.C. 28801-9801
Tel. (800) 522 – 4762

If hepatic detoxification abnormalities are detected :

MediClear® _____ Week 1: 1 scoop twice daily
_____ Week 2: 1 scoop three times each day
_____ Week 3: 1 scoop three times each day
_____ Week 4: 1 scoop one time daily

Silymarin _____ 200 mg - twice daily

After 4 weeks discontinue MediClear®, continue silymarin and begin
the standard **BrainRecovery.com** Parkinson's Protocol described
above.

MediClear® must be ordered by a *licensed health-care practitioner*
and is available from:

Thorne Research, Inc.
25820 Highway 2 West
PO Box 25
Dover, Idaho 83825
Tel. (800) 228-1966

**BrainSustain is a nutritional supplement designed to maintain
healthy brain function. It is not intended to treat or cure any
specific disease.**

References

1. *Living With Parkinson's Disease*, Kathleen E. Biziere, Matthias C. Kurth, Demos Vermande; ISBN: 1888799102   Published 1997
2. *Parkinson's : A Personal Story of Acceptance,*   Sandi Gordon, Lee W. Tempel,   Branden Publishing Co; ISBN: 0828319499; Published 1992
3. *Parkinson's Disease : The Complete Guide for Patients and Caregivers,* A. N. Lieberman(Editor), Frank L. Williams, Fireside; ISBN: 0671768190 ; Published 1993
4. *Understanding Parkinson's Disease : A Self Help Guide*, David L. Cram, Addicus Books ; ISBN: 0671768190 ; Published 1993

References

[1] Nutt, John G. In:Porter R.G. (ed), *100 Maxims in Neurology – (2) Parkinson's Disease*. St. Louis:Mosby Year Book, 1992: 1

[2] Parkinson's, James, An Essay on the Shaking Palsy. London Whittingham and Rowland,1817: 4

[3] Carlsson, A: The occurrence, distribution and physiological role of catecholamines in the nervous system. Pharmacol Rev 11:490-493, 1959

[4] Graham, D.G. Oxidative pathways for catecholamines in the genesis of neuromelanin and cytotoxic quinones. Mol Pharmacol 14:633-43, 1978

[5] Perry, T.L., Godin, D.V., Hansen, S.: Parkinson's disease: A disorder due to nigral glutathione deficiency? Neurosci Lett 33: 305-310, 1982

[6] Sechi, G., Deledda, M.G., Bua, G., et al., Reduced glutathione in the treatment of early Parkinson's disease. Prog Neuropsychopharmacol Biol Psychiatry 20(7): 1159-70,1996

[7] Bains, J. S., Shaw, C.A.: Neurodegenerative disorders in humans: the role of glutathione in oxidative stress-mediated neuronal death. Brain Res Brain Res Rev 25 (3): 335-58,1997

[8] Tanner, C.M., Liver Abnormalities in Parkinson's disease. Geriatrics 46 (1): 60-63, 1991

[9] Perlmutter, D., New Perspectives in Parkinson's Disease. Townsend Letter for Doctors 162: 48-50, 1997

[10] Vendemiale, G., Grattagliano, I., Altomare, E., et al., Effect of acetaminophen on hepatic glutathione compartmentation and mitochondrial energy metabolism in the rat. Biochem Pharmacol 25:52 (8): 1147-54, 1996

[11] Przedborski, S., Jackson-Lewia, V., Muthane, U., et al., Chronic levodopa administration alters mitochondrial respiratory chain activity. Ann Neurol 34 (5): 715-23, 1993

[12] Birkmayer, J.G. D., et al, Nicotinamide Adenine Dinucleotide (NADH) – A New Therapeutic Approach to Parkinson's Disease: Comparison of Oral and Parenteral Application. Acta Neurol Scand 87 (146): 32-35 1993

[13] Schults, C.W., Haas, R.H., Passov, D., Beal, M.F., Coenzyme Q10 Levels Correlate with the Activities of Complexes I and II/III in Mitochondria from Parkinsonian and Nonparkinsonian Subjects. Ann Neurol 42:261-264,1997

[14] Schults, C.W., Beal, M.F., Fontaine, K. et al., Absorption, tolerability and effects on mitochondrial activity of oral coenzyme Q10 in parkinsonian patients, Neurology 50: 793-795,1998

[15] Mortensen, S.A., Leth, A., Agner, E., Dose-related decrease of serum coenzyme Q10 during treatment with HMG-CoA reductase inhibitors. Mol Aspects of Med 18(Suppl.) S137-44, 1997

[16] Crook, T.H., Tinklenberg, J., Yesavage, J., et al., Effects of phosphatidylserine in age-associated memory impairment. Neurology 41:644-49, 1991

[17] Golbe, L.I., Farrell, T.M., David, P.H., Case-control study of early life dietary factors in Parkinson's disease. Arch Neurol 45(12): 1350-3, 1988

[18] Fahn, S., The endogenous toxin theory of the etiology of Parkinson's disease and a pilot trial of high-dose antioxidants in an attempt to slow the progression of the illness. Ann N Y Acad Sci 570:186-96, 1989

[19] Olanow, C.W., Attempts to obtain neuroprotection in Parkinson's disease. Neurololgy 49 (Suppl 1) S26-S33, 1997

[20] Pahan, K., Sheikh, G.S., Nmboodiri, A.M.S., et al., N-acetyl cysteine inhibits induction of NO production by endotoxin or cytokine stimulated rat peritoneal macrophages, C6 glial cells and astrocytes. Free Radical Biology and Medicine 24(1):39-48, 1998

[21] Steffen, V., Santiago, M., de la Cruz, C.P., et al, Effect of intraventricular injection of 1-methyl-4-phenylpyridinium protection by acetyl-L-carnitine. Human Exp Toxicol 14:865-871,1995

[22] Sato, Y., Kikuyama, M., Oizumi, K., High prevalence of vitamin D deficiency and reduced bone mass in Parkinson's disease. Neurology 49(5): 1273-78, 1997

[23] Sardar, S., Chakraborty, A., Chatterjee, M., Comparative effectiveness of vitamin D3 and dietary vitamin E on peroxidation of lipids and enzymes of the hepatic antioxidant system in Sprague-Dawley rats.Int J Vitam Nutr Res 66(1):39-45, 1996

[24] Wu, W.R., Zhu, X.Z., Involvement of monoamine oxidase inhibition in neuroprotective and neurorestorative effects of Ginkgo biloba extract against MPTP- induced nigrostriatal dopaminergic toxicity in C57 mice. Life Sci 65(2): 157-64, 1999

[25] Przedborski, S., Jackson-Lewis, V., Muthane, U., et al., Chronic levodopa administration alters cerebral mitochondrial respiratory chain activity. Ann Neurol 34 (5): 715-23, 1993

CHAPTER TWO

Multiple Sclerosis

Multiple sclerosis (MS) is a fairly common and generally progressive disease of the central nervous system with a prevalence in the United States of approximately 350,000 cases annually.[1] Although the onset of MS typically occurs between the ages of 10-59 years, onset as early as 2 years of age has been described.[2] Annual expenditures for the treatment of this disease in the United States exceed $2.5 billion.[3] While typically regarded as a cause of morbidity, more than 3,000 Americans die each year as a direct consequence of MS - a disease in which the cause has remained stubbornly elusive.[4]

The historical attempts to identify the cause of multiple sclerosis have been filled with bleak commentary. As Godfried Sonderdank, Court Physician of Schiedam, Holland, reported in the 14th century when describing a disease now thought to represent MS: "Believe me, there is no cure for this illness. It comes directly from God. Even Hippocrates and Gallenus would not be of any help here."[5]

Over a century ago, the genesis of multiple sclerosis was attributed to some form of infection. As the French physician Pierre Marie reported in his lectures of 1891:

"Before concluding this enumeration, a paragraph must be devoted to unnamed infections, so frequent, so little known, I might add so much disregarded. There are no special symptoms at the onset which indicate its existence; fever is known to have occurred, prolonged discomfort with or without gastrointestinal symptoms, occasionally jaundice or pulmonary trouble, nothing else being known about the disease. In such a case, gentlemen, you must not doubt that this is certainly a case of infection, but of a kind that it has not received any definite clinical name. As regards the patients in whom insular sclerosis (multiple sclerosis) seems to occur from the influence of injury or physical cause, my conviction is that these cases are also due to infection, but that the infection has passed away completely unperceived, while some less important but more dramatic incident has alone attracted the attention of the patient or those who are with him."[6]

By 1998, at least 16 infectious agents had been identified as possibly causing multiple sclerosis. Under strict scientific scrutiny, none has been found to specifically induce the disease.

But recently, the most convincing data ever presented relating infection with a specific organism to multiple sclerosis has been reported from the *Department of Neurology and Pathology, Vanderbilt School of Medicine, Nashville, Tennessee.* Dr. Subramaniam Sriram and co-workers, publishing their results in the July 1999 issue of *Annals of Neurology,* have demonstrated the presence of a specific type of bacteria in 100% of the 37 multiple sclerosis patients they studied. As the

> *By 1998, at least 16 infectious agents had been identified as possibly causing multiple sclerosis.*

authors reported, "The evidence of *Chlamydia pneumoniae* in both progressive MS and relapsing-remitting patients suggests that the infection of the central nervous system with *Chlamydia pneumoniae* occurs early and persists perhaps throughout the course of the disease and does not differentiate between different clinical subtypes of the disease."[7]

This organism, *Chlamydia pneumoniae,* is a fairly recent addition to the list of bacteria known to affect humans. It is now recognized as a cause of pneumonia, pharyngitis, bronchitis, and several chronic diseases. More importantly, *Chlamydia pneumoniae* has now been recognized as playing at least some causative role in reactive arthritis and coronary artery disease – medical conditions which, like MS, are characterized by ongoing inflammation.

The idea that multiple sclerosis may be caused by some form of infectious agent is supported by several interesting observations. On the Faroe Islands prior to 1920, MS was essentially unknown. Subsequent to the invasion of British troops, the incidence of MS increased dramatically.[8] This would support the contention that MS, at least on the Faroe Islands, was caused by some infectious agent to which the native population had not been previously exposed.

In addition, the cerebrospinal fluid (CSF) in patients with documented multiple sclerosis, is typically found to contain high amounts of specific proteins known to be elevated in other nervous system disorders in which infectious causes have been clearly identified.

If there is such a strong relationship between the presence of *Chlamydia pneumoniae* and multiple sclerosis, how could its presence have been missed by researchers for so many years? The answer lies in the fact that the discovery of *Chlamydia* in the spinal fluid of MS patients required the development of a very sophisticated test to detect a unique protein found on the cell wall of the *Chlamydia pneumoniae* organism itself. Indeed, this is not the first example of a profound delay in the identification of an elusive bacterium as the cause of a specific illness. It has been only in the past few years that the bacteria *Helicobactor pylori* has been demonstrated to be the causative agent in most cases of gastric ulcers. Incredibly, *Helicobactor pylori* has been identified in the stomachs of humans since the early 1900's, but medical researchers couldn't bring themselves to admit the possibility that a disease like gastric ulcers could be caused by a simple bacterium.

Another observation supporting the relationship between *Chlamydia pneumoniae* and multiple sclerosis is based on the discovery that two commonly used medications for multiple sclerosis, *interferon-beta* and *methotrexate,* profoundly inhibit the growth of the *Chlamydia* bacterium.[9] This is interesting and provocative information as we don't yet fully understand why these drugs are sometimes effective in MS treatment.

Over the past several years, the medical literature has published various articles describing specific viruses thought to be *the* causative agent for multiple sclerosis, only to have these reports subsequently refuted. But this new research describing the possible relationship between *Chlamydia pneumoniae* and multiple sclerosis is most compelling. And the good news is that unlike viruses, specific antimicrobial medicines are available to treat *Chlamydia pneumoniae*.

Based upon this research, it is not unreasonable for patients with multiple sclerosis to consider an empiric treatment for *Chlamydia pneumoniae*. As this discovery is so new, no specific treatment protocols have as yet been created. And it will likely be several years until clinical trials have been designed, approved, funded, completed, and ultimately published, until we know for sure that MS patients should be treated. But in light of the present evidence, empirically treating MS patients for *Chlamydia pneumoniae* seems reasonable. Obviously this decision be should discussed with the treating physician. Antibiotics generally quite effective in treating *Chlamydia pneumoniae* infections include **doxycycline** and **tetracycline**. Doxycycline may be the more effective treatment since it is more able to penetrate the blood-brain barrier to enter the brain.

Over the past two decades, well-respected researchers have described the possible link between various autoimmune diseases like multiple sclerosis and infection with the yeast *Candida albicans*. In his informative book *The Yeast Syndrome*, Dr. John Trowbridge discussed autoimmune diseases and stated "they appear to be among the growing number of otherwise unrelated disorders partially caused by inflammation and destruction of cells, tissues, and organs, by the body's own antibodies (auto-antibodies). These disorders belong to the autoimmune classification of diseases. Science has not explained why the body should lose the ability to distinguish between substances that are 'self' and those that are 'non-self'. An accumulating stack of evidence is pointing the finger of suspicion directly at *Candida albicans*, as well as other parasites or infections. How the yeast organism fosters a compromise of normal immune function is the subject of investigation and much speculation by the worldwide scientific and clinical communities."[10]

Because of the frequent association of Candidiasis (yeast overgrowth) with various autoimmune diseases like multiple sclerosis, we examined 10 adult MS patients for the presence of specific antibodies directed against *Candida albicans* as an indicator of infection or overgrowth of this specific form of yeast. Our published results indicated elevated levels of immunoglobulin (one of the body's immune proteins) against *Candida,* or *Candida* immune complexes (immunoglobulin bound to *Candida*) in 7 of the 10 patients evaluated.[11] (for the full text of this article visit: www.brainrecovery.com/msfatigue.htm

When elevated *Candida* immunoglobulins are found, our next step is to perform a *Comprehensive Digestive Stool Analysis* (CDSA) available from Great Smokies Diagnostic Laboratory (see below). This provides information not only indicating the amount of *Candida* overgrowth, but in addition describes which specific non-pharmaceutical and pharmaceutical agents would be useful for treatment.

In addition to the level of *Candida* overgrowth and sensitivity of a patient's *Candida* to various therapeutic agents, the CDSA provides other important information. *Lactobacillus acidophilus* is considered one of the "helpful bacteria" that normally resides in the gut. These symbiotic bacteria assist in assimilation of nutrients and produce various chemicals needed for maintenance of a healthy gut lining. In our 1995 study, 8 of 9 M.S. patients demonstrated significantly depressed levels of colonic *Lactobacillus* bacteria.[12] (See table 2.1)

The Dysbiosis Index is another bit of helpful information provided by the CDSA. The Dysbiosis Index essentially represents a ratio of potentially harmful bacteria divided by friendly or normal bacteria typically found in the gut, and therefore provides another indication of the status of gut health. In our study of 9 MS patients, 100% demonstrated an abnormally high Dysbiosis Index.

patient	1	2	3	4	5	6	7	8	9
Lactobaccilus (normal 2+ or greater)	0	2+	0	0	0	0	0	0	1+
Dysbiosis Index (normal 0-3)	10	6	8	6	6	16	6	12	8

Table 2.1 Lactobacillus count and Dysbiosis index in 9 multiple sclerosis patients as determined by CDSA stool analysis.
From: Perlmutter, D., Fatigue in Multiple Sclerosis. Townsend Letter for Doctors 1995 [11]

Dysbiosis, an imbalance of gut bacteria, is commonly recognized in patients suffering from inflammatory diseases of the bowel. How this specifically relates to multiple sclerosis was elegantly described in a report appearing in the highly respected medical journal, *The Lancet*. This study, also published in 1995, evaluated the frequency of brain MRI changes like those seen in multiple sclerosis (white matter plaques) in patients with inflammatory bowel disease compared to normal non-afflicted individuals. The results of this study were profound. Hyper-intense, focal, white-matter lesions ranging from 2 – 8 mm in diameter were seen in 20 of 48 patients (42%) with Crohn's disease (an inflammatory condition of the bowel), and in 11 of 24 patients (46%) with ulcerative colitis (another inflammatory bowel condition). These were patients who *didn't have MS* or any other nervous system disease, just bowel inflammation. And yet, their MRI scans were identical to those of patients with documented MS! Abnormalities in the white matter were seen in only 8 of 50 (16%) healthy volunteers. As the authors reported: "The frequency of focal white matter lesions in patients with inflammatory bowel disease is almost as high as that in patient's with multiple sclerosis."[13]

"The frequency of focal white matter lesions in patients with inflammatory bowel disease is almost as high as that in patient's with multiple sclerosis."

These findings provide convincing evidence supporting the relationship between gut abnormalities and brain pathology.

One of the central tenants of holistic medicine holds that there is an important relationship between all of the body's systems. Thus, focusing exclusively on controlling the immune system in the brain seems somewhat narrow-minded. New research clearly reveals a very important relationship between MS and problems in the digestive system like inflammatory bowel disease, yeast overgrowth, and low levels of healthful bacteria (*Lactobacillus acidophillus*). Focusing exclusively on the nervous system with MRI scans and spinal fluid analysis shortchanges the healthcare provider's ability to gain a more comprehensive understanding of many other factors that may underlie the overactivation of the immune system.

Dietary Keys

For many years it has been known that there is a progressive increase in incidence of multiple sclerosis with increasing latitude both north and south of the equator. For example, the incidence of multiple sclerosis is 6–14 per 100,000 in the southern United States and southern Europe, and progressively increases to 80 per 100,000 in the northern United States, northern Europe, and Canada. A similar gradient exists in the Southern Hemisphere and is well recognized in Australia and New Zealand.[14]

Researchers have attempted to explain this striking geographic distribution, but as yet no definitive explanation has been offered although such ideas as an "environmental factor" or a "virus" are frequently offered in textbooks.

But there are some interesting exceptions to the north/south distribution of multiple sclerosis cases. Countries like China, Japan, and Korea, while at a similar latitude as the United States and various European countries, have a much lower incident rate of multiple sclerosis. Taking a look at just one northern country, Norway, reveals that prevalence of multiple sclerosis actually varies quite dramatically in various districts just within that country. Researcher Roy L. Swank, M.D., Ph.D., provided an important observation when he published research in 1952 showing that there was a direct correlation between the incidence of multiple sclerosis in various districts in Norway and the amount of dairy products consumed by the population of those specific regions.[15] This important, but for the most part unrecognized discovery offered the first meaningful explanation as to why MS is so common in some areas and almost unheard of in others. Since populations living in colder climates tend to consume diets higher in fat compared to those living in more tropical regions, Doctor Swank's theory was the first to explain the north-south distribution of MS.

Countries like Japan, Korea, and China have, until just recently, consumed diets far lower in fat than countries with high rates of MS, like the United States, Canada, and most of northern Europe. The direct relationship between MS mortality and dietary fat, especially saturated fats and animal fats was eloquently described in an extensive study involving 36 countries appearing in the *American Journal of Epidemiology* in 1995.[16] In a comprehensive review article appearing in the highly respected peer review journal *Neurology*, author Klaus Lauer, M.D. stated: " When the important principle of consistency is applied, however, several traits can be delineated. Both on a global scale and within smaller geographic units, the MS rate was significantly correlated repeatedly with one or another parameter reflecting the consumption of animal fat, animal protein, and meat from non-marine mammals…"[17] Unfortunately, while subsequent studies have continued to explore and confirm Swank's original hypothesis, the concept that nutrition plays any significant role in multiple sclerosis has not yet really gained a foothold in modern western medical thinking. Indeed in a recent review article entitled *Management of Multiple Sclerosis* appearing in the prestigious *New*

MS rate was significantly correlated repeatedly with one or another parameter reflecting the consumption of animal fat.

England Journal of Medicine, the authors presented an overview of what they felt was the state of the art in treatment options for M.S.. Every pharmaceutical therapy from steroids to interferon, to powerful chemotherapy drugs were presented without a single mention of nutritional intervention.[18]

Multiple sclerosis, like many other diseases of modern civilization, is a disease quite simply caused by an overactive and misdirected immune system. For reasons that remain unclear, the immune system reacts against protective insulating cover (myelin) of the nerves of the central nervous system and in addition causes damage to the actual nerve body (axon). White blood cells called *lymphocytes* attack myelin as if it were some invading organisms or foreign substance. When the body's immune system fails to control itself and lymphocytes attack normal body tissue, the disease process that ensues is called an *autoimmune* disease. Other autoimmune diseases include rheumatoid arthritis, systemic lupus erythematosus (SLE) and even some forms of vascular disease.

The mainstay of modern western medical treatment for autoimmune diseases involves the administration of *immunosuppressive drugs,* designed to reduce the activity of the immune system in a general way. Indeed, this remains the focal point of treatment for acute flare-ups of multiple sclerosis. Unfortunately, these potent drugs like *cortisone, prednisone, methotrexate* and *cytoxan,* reduce the effectiveness of the *entire* immune system, and are fraught with other, sometimes life threatening, side effects.

In multiple sclerosis, lymphocytes somehow receive inappropriate signals directing them to attack the brain and spinal cord. But what are the messages which normally control lymphocytes? Their activity is regulated by a group of chemicals called *prostaglandins,* so named as they were originally isolated from the prostate gland. Prostaglandins can be conveniently divided into three main groups: PG-1, PG-2, and PG-3. These three groups of prostaglandins are all derived from a special type of dietary fat called *essential fatty acids,* or EFA's. EFA's are not produced in the body and hence are called essential because our survival depends on adequate nutritional sources of these critical nutrients. The two EFA's important in the production of prostaglandins are linolenic acid and linoleic acid, part of the omega 3 and omega 6 fatty acid groups, respectively.

The role of prostaglandins from groups 1 and 3 is to moderate or tone down immune activity and inflammation. Prostaglandins in group 2 on the other hand signal the lymphocytes to become more active in the immune response and induce inflammatory activity. In normal situations a healthy balance is achieved in immune function. Under the influence of prostaglandins from the PG-2 group, the white blood cells are activated, but this activity is kept in check by prostaglandins from groups 1 and 3. Interestingly, the cerebrospinal fluid, a liquid covering the brain and spinal cord, has been shown to contain significantly less linoleic acid in multiple sclerosis patients compared to controls. Linoleic acid is the precursor to the Prostaglandin 1 group, so its deficiency could allow overactivation of the immune system.

With the understanding that prostaglandins 1 and 3 calm the immune system while prostaglandin 2 is pro-inflammatory, the epidemiological studies describing diet and risk for MS make sense. Thus, diets rich in vegetables, nuts, seeds and fish, being good sources of linolenic and linoleic acids, favor the production of prostaglandins 1 and 3, and are associated with lower rates of MS. Diets based on animal fats, dairy products and animal proteins favor prostaglandin 2 formation and are associated with higher rates of MS, more frequent exacerbations, and higher MS related mortality rates.[19] It is this relationship between animal fat and immune activation that explains the observations made by Dr. Swank over 40 years ago.

What emerges from this simplified description of the regulation of the activity of lymphocytes is that it may be possible to reduce the overactivity of immune function in multiple sclerosis by providing dietary sources of linoleic and linolenic acids, producing more of the "good prostaglandins" – groups 1 and 3. This approach to MS treatment has been followed for decades in Europe and in various

Scandinavian countries where clinicians have long supported the use of EFA supplementation not only to treat the symptoms of multiple sclerosis, but also to reduce the frequency of new events.

The reluctance of American doctors to employ essential fatty acid supplements flies in the face of substantial high quality research supporting their use appearing regularly in our best journals. Indeed, after a comprehensive review of the current research on the subject, *Columbia University*'s Dr. Robert Dworkin recently stated in the journal *Neurology*: "The impetus for these studies was a series of reports of a deficiency of linoleic acid in the serum of patients with multiple sclerosis, as well as epidemiological data indicating an association between dietary essential fatty acids and the prevalence of M.S....We have reanalyzed the data from three double-blind trials of linoleic acid in the treatment of MS. Our most important finding is that patients with minimal or no disability at entry had a significantly smaller increase in disability over the course of the trials than did control patients. Additional analyses indicated that patients with minimal or no disability who were treated with linoleic acid did not have a significant change from the beginning of treatment to the end of the trial, whereas control patients had a significant increase in disability."[20]

When physicians read medical journals, most of the information they retain comes not from the articles but from the advertisements.

In the U.S. it is rare to find a physician who feels comfortable including essential fatty acid supplements in an MS program, especially in the face of the multi-billion dollar expenditure on the part of pharmaceutical companies to convince doctors that drugs are the only answer. Unfortunately, as has been shown by *Harvard* researcher Jerry Avorn, when physicians read medical journals, most of the information they retain comes not from the articles but from the advertisements.[21]

Any multiple sclerosis sufferer who has explored nutritional approaches to this illness has likely discovered frequent reference to *evening primrose oil*. The healing power of the evening primrose plant has been known for centuries. It was used by Native Americans for infections and a variety of skin conditions. Over the past half century, this special oil has been widely recommended in Europe as a nutritional supplement helpful in the treatment of multiple sclerosis.

But what is it about evening primrose oil that makes it so useful in MS and other autoimmune diseases? Analysis of this oil reveals that it is a very rich source of linoleic acid which, as described above, is an essential fatty acid and the precursor of prostaglandin 1 - critically important in controlling the immune system. Other rich sources of linoleic acid are *borage oil* and *black current seed oil*. These supplements are nonprescription items, widely available in health food stores. When buying any of these oils, read labels to determine the content of *GLA* - the metabolite of linoleic acid that directly influences the production of prostaglandin 1.

Prostaglandin 3 is also very important in reducing the overactive immune response in multiple sclerosis. While much less potent than prostaglandin 1, it nevertheless plays an important role by reducing the activity of inflammation enhancing prostaglandin 2. Prostaglandin 3 is derived from the other essential fatty acid, linolenic acid, which can also be supplemented in the diet. Oil of flaxseed, for example, is 50% to 60% linolenic acid. But in order to complete the process of PG-3 production, linolenic acid must first be converted to 2 important intermediate fatty acids, *EPA* and *DHA*. The conversion of linolenic acid to EPA and then to DHA is actually a fairly inefficient process. It has been estimated that under the best of circumstances humans convert only about 2.7% of administered linolenic acid to EPA. Dietary saturated fat and cholesterol reduce this conversion. In addition, the final step, converting EPA to DHA, requires a specific enzyme that may not function appropriately in a large segment of the population. So even though an individual may be taking a supplemental oil providing an adequate source of linolenic acid, it may not be contributing much of a therapeutic benefit.

But here's the good news. Various fish oil products are available which are rich in preformed EPA and DHA eliminating the concern about the effectiveness of linolenic acid conversion. Consumption of EPA/ DHA containing fish may explain why Eskimos, who should be considered at high risk for MS because they live at far northern latitudes, hardly ever get the disease, or other autoimmune diseases for that matter. EPA/DHA supplements, like the sources of GLA described above, should be kept refrigerated to keep them from becoming rancid.

Now let's focus on prostaglandin 2, which you'll recall enhances inflammation and immune activity. There are dietary habits that will increase production of prostaglandin 2, and may therefore prove detrimental in multiple sclerosis. Perhaps the biggest trigger of prostaglandin 2 production is dietary fat, especially saturated

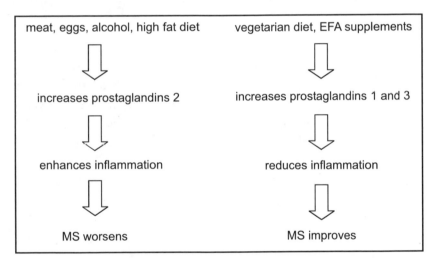

Figure 2.1. The role of prostaglandins in M.S.

fats and cholesterol (animal fats). Alcohol further enhances PG-2 production while less is produced in a diet supplemented with zinc, vitamin C, vitamins B3 and B6, and a good source of EPA/DHA (see figure 2.1).

This is why a low-fat, essentially vegetarian diet is *critical* for the multiple sclerosis patient. In one study following 146 patients for an average of 17 years on a very low-fat diet, MS was noted to progress much less rapidly in comparison to patients not fat-restricted. There was also a significant reduction of mortality as well as frequency and severity of exacerbations of MS in the fat-restricted group. As Dr. Swank indicated, "if treated early in the disease, before significant disability had developed, a high percentage of cases remain unchanged for up to 20 years."[22]

Creating the most advantageous environment for repair and regeneration of myelin requires an adequate supply of EFA's.

Finally, about 75% of myelin is composed of fat, with a substantial amount coming from the essential fatty acids. Creating the most advantageous environment for repair and regeneration of myelin requires an adequate supply of EFA's along with other cofactors like vitamin B12 (see below).

Nutritionists, naturopaths, chiropractors, and holistically oriented medical doctors have for years been treating multiple sclerosis with essential fatty acid supplements, vitamins, and minerals, and fat-restricted diets, and have been doing so with great success. This approach to MS is founded on the principle of strengthening the body, working with nature, and not fighting a war using the patient as a battleground as is the case with the use of potent immunosuppressive drugs.

Antioxidant Protection

Vitamin D

Here's another reason why MS may be more prevalent in northern latitudes. Sunshine. Living further from the equator reduces the amount of sun exposure an individual may receive. Sun exposure is responsible for the formation of the active form of vitamin D which we now know has powerful antioxidant properties. That means vitamin D, like the more familiar antioxidant vitamins C, E, and lipoic acid, helps to reduce the activity of damaging *free radicals* – chemicals used by the immune system to destroy tissue.

In MS, increased activity of free radicals destroys the myelin covering over the nerve cells. This is why antioxidants are key players in the nutritional part of a comprehensive MS program, and why vitamin D must now be included on the list.

More support for its use comes from two observations. First, as described above, MS rates are lower in populations eating cold water fish – a rich source of Vitamin D.

Second, in a recent publication in the journal *Neurology*, researchers demonstrated that on average, MS patients are severely vitamin D deficient. Unfortunately, after making this discovery, the main conclusion reached by this study's authors was that because MS patients have low vitamin D levels, health care providers should watch for osteoporosis. The important antioxidant properties of vitamin D and its relevance to M.S. was completely overlooked.[23]

Finally, vitamin D has been shown to completely prevent the development of a multiple sclerosis-like disease (EAE) in the mouse model.[24] It is this model which has been used in the development of virtually all of the pharmaceutical preparations now advocated for MS treatment. It is interesting that the severity of EAE in mice is markedly reduced by linoleic acid, adding further support to its use (see above).

Vitamin E

Like vitamin D, vitamin E is fat-soluble and freely supports the regeneration of other brain antioxidants like vitamin C, and glutathione. Adequate supplementation with vitamin E is mandatory when essential fatty acids are used to keep these delicate oils from becoming oxidized - a process which renders them therapeutically useless.

Alpha Lipoic acid

As discussed in the introduction, alpha lipoic is emerging as one of the most powerful brain antioxidants available. Readily entering the sanctuary of the brain, lipoic acid is a critically important nutrient in all the neurodegenerative disorders. Assisting in the regeneration of other brain antioxidants, alpha lipoic acid is a key nutrient in the BrainRecovery.com protocol for M.S.

Ginkgo biloba

The antioxidant power of this ancient herb is now widely recognized. Ginkgo is useful in virtually all the neurodegenerative conditions due not only to its ability to reduce the activity of free radicals, but also because of its potent effects enhancing *neurotransmission*, the process by which neurons are able to communicate with each other.

N-acetyl-cysteine (NAC)

By enhancing the production of glutathione, one of the most important brain antioxidants, NAC is a key supplement in M.S. and all other neurodegenerative conditions. As yet, there is no preformed glutathione available for oral consumption that can produce any meaningful increase in blood glutathione levels. This can be accomplished with intravenous glutathione injection as described in the treatment of Parkinson's disease (see chapter one). Fortunately, orally administered NAC does lead to a significant increase in glutathione, hence its inclusion in the BrainRecovery.com M.S. protocol.

Cellular Energetics

Vitamin B12

The general lack of use of vitamin B12 in the treatment of MS by American physicians parallels their underutilization of the essential fatty acids. Vitamin B12, like essential fatty acids, cannot be patented. So it can't become an object of expensive advertising efforts in medical journals. Yet support for the use of vitamin B12 in MS treatment goes back at least to the 1950's. In 1957 German researchers published data demonstrating profound deficiencies of vitamin B12 in the blood of MS patients. Their results have been repeatedly confirmed with more recent medical publications showing low B12 levels not only in the blood, but also in the cerebrospinal fluid (CSF) of patients with MS.[25]

One of the most important functions of vitamin B12 in humans is its role in the formation and maintenance of myelin – that all-important insulating covering over nerves of the central nervous system. Multiple sclerosis is a disease characterized by myelin destruction as a consequence of an unregulated immunological reaction. Vitamin B12 deficiency not only enhances the destruction of myelin during an MS attack, but can also compromise the body's ability to repair the damaged myelin after the storm of destruction has subsided.

In addition to the important role of this vitamin in the formation, maintenance and repair of myelin, B12 has a direct stabilizing effect on the immune system. Thus, deficiency of vitamin B12 renders an individual more vulnerable to the damaging effects of overactivity of the immune system – the fundamental flaw in multiple sclerosis.

In an excellent review article entitled, "Multiple Sclerosis and Vitamin B12 Metabolism" published in the *Journal of Neuroimmunology*, Dr. E. H. Reynolds of King's College Hospital in London emphasized the importance of performing a *functional* evaluation of vitamin B12 in the evaluation of MS patients.[26] The test he described is a simple measurement of a chemical, *homocysteine*, normally found in the blood. One of the functions of B12 is to keep homocysteine levels in the normal range. An elevated level of homocysteine may indicate that B12, while present in normal amounts on blood testing, may still be functionally deficient. Physicians may balk at prescribing B12 injections for MS patients with normal blood B12 levels. That's why it's important to take it a step further and request a blood test for homocysteine. If elevated (over 10 µmol/L) your physician may feel justified in administering B12.

Almost universally our patients have felt increased energy and a better sense of wellbeing soon after beginning B12 injections. That's not surprising given the fact that B12 participates in so many chemical processes in the body dealing with energy production. In fact, combining B12 injections with oral NADH, another health food store supplement, provides a powerful antidote for the generalized fatigue that so frequently plagues MS patients. NADH acts as a cofactor for cellular energy production. The usual adult dose of NADH is 5mg twice a day, usually taken first thing in the morning and at mid-day on an empty stomach.

Deficiency of vitamin B12 renders an individual more vulnerable to the damaging effects of overactivity of the immune system.

Phosphatidylserine

Lecithin has for decades been part of complementary treatment programs for M.S., and with good reason. Lecithin is one of the important building blocks for neuronal membranes, the real business end of brain cells where cell to cell communication takes place. Deficiencies of intracellular communication are the ultimate functional flaws in M.S.. Newer research has revealed that perhaps the most important component of lecithin is phosphatidylserine.

Thus, adequate amounts of phosphatidylserine are required not only to preserve, but also enhance the ability of nerves to transmit information.

Phosphatidylserine plays a major role in preserving function of the membrane surrounding the energy producing apparatus of the cell, the *mitochondria*. Inadequacies of function of the mitochondrial membrane compromise energy production and thus threatens the viability of the neuron.

Coenzyme Q10   (CoQ10)

Finally, the critical role of adequate CoQ10 in facilitating cellular energy production cannot be overstated. Also known as *ubiquinone* because of its ubiquitous presence in all living cells, inadequacies of CoQ10 threatens the fundamental process of cellular energy production and enhances the damaging effects of naturally occurring free radicals.

Hyperbaric Oxygen – Potent MS Therapy

Hyperbaric Oxygen Therapy (HBOT) is without question the most exciting innovation in the treatment of MS available today. Although seemingly new on the scene, medical literature citations attesting to the effectiveness of HBOT in treating MS date back some 30 years.

Clinicians in the United States remained completely in the dark about this powerful MS therapy until 1983. In that year an article entitled "Hyperbaric Oxygen as a Treatment of Multiple Sclerosis" appeared in the highly respected *New England Journal of Medicine*. This report detailed the results of a 1-year study evaluating the clinical course of a group of MS patients receiving HBOT (twenty, 90-minute treatments) compared to a similar group of MS patients without the treatment. The results were remarkable. Worsening of symptoms was observed in 55% of the untreated group, while only 12% of the patients treated with hyperbaric oxygen experienced a deterioration of function. Even more dramatic was the observation that many of the treated patients actually experienced *improvements* in a variety of symptoms including mobility, fatigability, tremor, bladder control, and visual symptoms. And to satisfy those who may choose to criticize the data, rest assured the study was randomized, double-blinded, and placebo-controlled.[27]

The publication of this report created an immediate sensation. While MS patients began demanding HBOT treatment, physicians recoiled at the prospect that a non-drug therapy could prove more effective than any of the pharmaceutical approaches they had come to rely on. This prompted medical researchers to perform a much more extensive study of HBOT's purported effectiveness in MS therapy.

Worsening of symptoms was observed in 55% of the untreated group, while only 12% of the patients treated with hyperbaric oxygen experienced a deterioration of function.

In 1987 the long awaited follow-up study was completed. Evaluating triple the number of patients and using the same treatment parameters, this research, published in the *Journal of Neurology, Neurosurgery, and Psychiatry,* not only confirmed the results of the original report, but, in addition, revealed a striking preservation of cerebellar function (coordination) in the HBOT treatment group compared to controls.[28]

Despite these and subsequent studies attesting to HBOT's effectiveness in MS therapy, with the exception of a handful of pioneering souls, American physicians have continued to turn their backs on hyperbaric oxygen. Fortunately this has not been the case for most of the rest of the world.

Perhaps the largest experience in treating MS with HBOT is taking place in the United Kingdom. There, the *Federation of MS Therapy Centres* operates 56 hyperbaric oxygen facilities and has compiled data evaluating the progress of some 10,000 MS patients over the past 14 years. Their protocol consists of an initial course of 20 treatments over 4 weeks, followed by a single treatment on a weekly basis thereafter. Over 1 million treatments have been administered, and all without a single serious complication.

Their published results offer a direct challenge to the overall pessimistic prognoses given to MS patients in the US. Patients were evaluated on the *Kurtzke* scale – a measure of overall functional ability used as a standard for evaluating the progress of MS patients worldwide. None of the patients with relapsing/remitting MS who had received at least 8 treatments every 3 months experienced any deterioration on the Kurtzke scale. In fact, 40% of these patients actually *improved* in functional ability with treatment.[29] For the full text of this study, visit: www.BrainRecovery.com/msfed.htm

What explains oxygen's profound benefit in multiple sclerosis? Oxygen delivered under pressure has some important physiological effects. In the animal model of multiple sclerosis, EAE, hyperbaric oxygen has been found to act as an immunosuppressive agent. That is, it reduces the overactivity of the immune system much like the many popular MS drugs, but without their dangerous side effects.[30]

Second, by improving local tissue oxygenation, the breakdown of myelin characteristic of the immune reaction is diminished. In addition, enhanced tissue oxygenation creates a more favorable environment for myelin repair, especially in conjunction with essential fatty acids and vitamin B12.

Third, hyperbaric oxygen has been demonstrated to improve the function of the *blood-brain barrier* – a layer of tightly packed cells which functions to exclude potentially dangerous substances from the sanctuary of the brain.[31] Deficiencies of the blood-brain barrier are common in MS.

Hyperbaric oxygen has been demonstrated to improve the function of the blood-brain barrier.

Case Report

R.R. is a pleasant 40 year old gentleman who was diagnosed with multiple sclerosis some 14 years ago. Despite vigorous pharmaceutical interventions, he suffered an almost relentless downhill course, confining him to a wheelchair and making him almost totally dependent on others for his day to day requirements of self care. After several months of treatment with hyperbaric oxygen therapy, his arm and leg strength improved and he regained the ability to walk with an assistive device. He writes:

> Dear Dr. Perlmutter:
>
> Regarding my positive results from hyperbaric oxygen therapy, I have noticed an improvement in energy with increased strength in my arms and less tremors in my hands. I am able to do more exercising such as sit-ups and lifting 5-pound weights. <u>One very important thing to me</u> is that my voice is stronger.
>
> At the start of hyperbaric therapy I used a wheelchair. Now I can use the walker for most things, except for long distances. Hyperbaric therapy is relaxing, and the solitude helps with my concentration.
>
> Thank you,
>
> R.R.

Fortunately, there are a growing number of facilities around the U.S. where multiple sclerosis patients can receive hyperbaric oxygen therapy. More about hyperbaric oxygen therapy can be found in chapter nine or visit www.BrainRecovery.com.

BrainRecovery.com –MS Summary

Diet

The MS diet is essentially vegetarian. Meat products and eggs enhance the formation of inflammation producing fatty acids. Protein sources include cold water fish and vegetable protein including soy products like tofu and soy protein powder. Dairy products should be minimized. Instead, choose soy-based cheeses and soy milk instead of cow's milk. Nuts, seeds and dark green leafy vegetables, all rich in essential fatty acids, should be emphasized. Alcohol should be eliminated since it enhances the formation of the damaging 2 series prostaglandins. When considering the possible cardiovascular benefits of alcohol, recognize that the MS diet with the supplements described below represents a potent program to reduce coronary artery disease risk. Read food product labels and reduce total fat, especially saturated fats.

Essential Fatty Acids (EFA'S) A good source of linolenic acid is flaxseed oil. But remember, the reason for taking a linolenic acid supplement is to assist your body in the manufacturing of DHA. Since this process may be inefficient, choose products with pre-formed DHA like many of the EPA/DHA fish oil supplements found in health food stores. Total daily DHA dosage should be in the range of 500 mg.

The strength of the linoleic acid supplement is determined by the GLA content. Total daily GLA dosage should approximate 300mg. Oil supplements should always be refrigerated and taken in conjunction with a daily dose of at least 200 IU of high quality vitamin E to keep them from degrading.

Vitamin B12.   Vitamin B12 is inexpensive and safe. Orally administered B12 is unable to achieve the therapeutic levels necessary for MS treatment. It must be given by injection. Our treatment protocol for vitamin B12 in adult MS patients begins with a daily injection of 1000 mcg (1 cc) of vitamin B12 (cyanocobalamin) for 5 consecutive days followed by one injection twice weekly thereafter. Our patients are almost always able to learn how to administer these intramuscular injections themselves, generally finding the front of the thigh muscle to be the easiest injection site. Pateints should receive instructions for this injection from a physician, nurse, or other qualified healthcare provider. It's a good idea to alternate legs one injection to the next.

Vitamin D. Daily dose 400 IU. Often this will be found in combination with vitamin A and/or some form of fish oil. These combinations are fine. If combined with fish oil, check the amount of DHA as this may allow a reduction of the DHA supplement.

Other Nutrients. Vitamins B3, B6, and vitamin C, as well as the minerals zinc and magnesium reduce the formation of the inflammation producing prostaglandin 2. Critically important antioxidants to reduce the damaging effects of free radicals generated during MS attacks include alpha lipoic acid, vitamin E, vitamin C, NAC, and Ginkgo biloba. Enhancing cellular metabolism requires adequate phosphatidylserine, coenzyme Q10, and NADH. With the exception of sufficient alpha lipoic acid and injectable vitamin B12, appropriate amounts of all of these vitamins and nutrients are found in the Brain Sustain™ supplement.

Chlamydia pneumoniae

It is very likely that this bacterium is related to MS. So it makes sense to consider empiric antibiotic treatment for *Chlamydia pneumoniae* using doxycycline. Our protocol for the empiric treatment of *Chlamydia pneumoniae* in our M.S. patients is:

Doxycycline 100 mg twice a day for 14 days

Again, the decision to engage in this empiric treatment should be made after patient and physician consider the literature linking *Chlamydia pneumoniae* to multiple sclerosis, as well as the potential risks of taking a course of doxycycline or other antibiotic. It is always important when taking any antibiotic to also use a *probiotic*. These are nutritional supplements designed to reestablish appropriate levels of the "friendly bacteria" in the gut like *Lactobacillus acidophilus* and others which aid in the absorption of nutrients, help maintain the integrity of the gut lining, and assist in detoxification (see below).

Candida

This organism has been associated with hyperimmune diseases and specifically MS. To check for *Candida*, have your doctor order a *Comprehensive Digestive Stool Analysis* (CDSA) from Great Smokies Diagnostic Laboratory (tel. 800-522-4762). If *Candida* is found, the CDSA will provide a list of appropriate treatments. *Candida albicans* is almost always sensitive to the drug **fluconazole**, but be certain your physician checks the sensitivity results on the CDSA. A typical adult dosage for fluconazole (Diflucan®) is 100mg daily for 14 days, followed by 100mg every other day for another 14 days. This means that 21 tablets will be taken during the 4-week treatment. Other treatments may be indicated by the results of the CDSA. If low *Lactobacillus acidophilus* is found, add a supplement like Kyo-Dophilus®. Each tablet supplies 1 billion *Lactobacillus acidophilus* organisms. Take 1-3 tablets daily on an empty stomach with non-chlorinated water.

Hyperbaric Oxygen Therapy

See text this chapter, chapter nine, and visit **www.BrainRecovery.com**.

BrainRecovery.com
Multiple Sclerosis Protocol

Vitamin B12 _____ 1cc (1000mcg) injected IM daily
for 5 days, then twice weekly (see above)

Essential fatty acids   <u>daily dose</u>
   Linolenic acid
      EPA / DHA fish oil providing _____ DHA 500 mg
      (see note below)
  and,

   Linoleic acid
      Evening Primrose oil, or
      Borage oil, or
      Black Currant oil providing _____ GLA 300 mg

Vitamins and Antioxidants

Vitamin B3	50 mg
Vitamin B6	50 mg
Vitamin C	400 mg
Vitamin E	200 IU
Vitamin D	200 IU
Ginkgo biloba	30 mg
Alpha lipoic acid	100 mg
N-Acetyl Cysteine	200 mg

Cellular Energizers

Coenzyme Q10 _____ 30 mg
NADH _____ 5 mg (twice)
Phosphatidylserine _____ 50 mg

Minerals

Magnesium _____ 200 mg
Zinc _____ 10 mg

Or, if using the Brain Sustain™ supplement:

Essential Fatty Acids, B12 and NADH as above, and :

Brain Sustain™ _____ 1 scoop daily

Alpha Lipoic Acid _____ 60 mg per day

Note:

The highest quality DHA containing fish oil supplements are manufactured by **Nordic Naturals, Inc.,** and are available by calling *i* **Nutritionals** at: 1-800-530-1982 or by visiting the website www.BrainRecovery.com

BrainSustain is a nutritional supplement designed to maintain healthy brain function. It is not intended to treat or cure any specific disease.

Resources

1. *Multiple sclerosis – A Self-help guide to Its Management.* By Judy Graham, 1989, Inner Traditions Intl Ltd; ISBN: 0892812427
2. *The Multiple Sclerosis Diet Book : A Low-Fat Diet for the Treatment of M.S.* by Roy L. Swank, Barbara Brewer Dugan. 1987, Doubleday ; ISBN: 0385232799
3. *Multiple Sclerosis : Over 100 Recipes to Help Control Symptoms (Recipes for Health)* by Geraldine Fitzgerald, Fenella Briscoe 1998, Thorsons Pub; ISBN: 0722531427
4. *Women Living With Multiple Sclerosis* by Judith Lynn Nichols, 1999, Hunter House; ISBN: 0897932188
5. *Smart Fats* by Michael A. Scmidt, 1997, Frog, Ltd; ISBN1-883319-62-5

References

[1] Rudnick, R.A., Ransohoff, R.M., Herndon, R.M., Multiple Sclerosis and Other Myelin Disorders. In *Clinical Neurology Volume 3*, Joint, R.J.(ed.), Rochester, New York, Lippincott Williams & Wilkins, p.9, 1998

[2] Bejar, J.M., Zieglar, D.K., Onset of Multiple Sclerosis in a 24-Month Child. Arch Neurol 41:881-82, 1984

[3] Anderson, D.W., Ellenberg, J.H., Leventhat, C.M., et al., Revised estimate of the prevalence of multiple sclerosis in the United States. Ann Neurol 31: 333-36, 1992

[4] Ibid.

[5] Medaer, R., Does the History of Multiple Sclerosis Go Back as Far as the Fourteenth Century? Acta Neurol Scand 60:189-92, 1979

[6] Marie, P., *Lectures on Diseases of the Spinal Cord*, Lubbock, M. (trans). London, New Sydenham Society, 153:134-136, 1895

[7] Sriram, S., Stratton, C.W., Yao, S., et al., *Chlamydia pneumoniae* Infection of the Central Nervous System in Multiple Sclerosis. Ann Neurol 46: 6-14, 1999

[8] 3(33): 11

[x9] Sriram, S., Stratton, C.W., Yao, S., et al., *Chlamydia pneumoniae* Infection of the Central Nervous System in Multiple Sclerosis. Ann Neurol 46: 6-14, 1999

[10] Trowbridge, J., Walker, M., *The Yeast Syndrome*. Bantam Books, New York, P.35, 1988

[11] Perlmutter, D., Fatigue in Multiple Sclerosis. Townsend Letter for Doctors 148: 48-50, 1995

[12] Ibid.

[13] Geissler, A., Andus, T., Roth, M., et al., Focal white-matter lesions of the brain in patients with inflammatory bowel disease. Lancet 345: 897-98, 1995

[14] Rudnick, R.A., Ransohoff,R.M., Herndon, R.M., Multiple Sclerosis and Other Myelin Disorders. In *Clinical Neurology Volume 3*, Joint, R.J.(ed.), Rochester, New York, Lippincott Williams & Wilkins, p.9, 1998

[15] Swank, R.L., Lerstad, O., Strom, A., Multiple sclerosis in rural Norway: its geographic and occupational incidence in relation to nutrition. N Eng J Med 246:721-28, 1952

[16] Esparza, M.L., Sasaki, S., Kesteloot, H., Nutrition, latitude and multiple sclerosis mortality: an ecologic study. Am J Epidemiol 142(7): 733-77, 1995

[17] Lauer, K., Diet and multiple sclerosis. Neurology 49(Suppl 2): S55-S61, 1997

[18] Rudick, R.A., Cohen, J.A. Weinstock-Guttman, B., et al., Management of Multiple Sclerosis. N Eng J Med337(22):1604-67, 1997

[19] Esparza, M.L., Sasaki, S., Kesteloot, H., Nutrition, latitude and multiple sclerosis mortality: an ecologic study. Am J Epidemiol 142(7): 733-77, 1995

[20] Dworkin, R.H., Bates, D., Millar, J.H.D., et al., Linoleic acid and multiple sclerosis: A reanalysis of three double-blind trials. Neurology 34:1441-45, 1984

[21] Avorn, J., In: *Pushing Drugs to Doctors.* Consumer Reports,Feb.: p 88,1992

[22] Swank, R.S., Multiple sclerosis: the lipid relationship. A J Clin Nutr 48: 1387-93, 1988

[23] Nieves, J., Cosman, F., Shen, H.J. et al., High prevalence of vitamin D deficiency and reduced bone mass in multiple sclerosis. Neurology 44(9): 1687-92, 1994

[24] Hayes, C.E., Cantorna, M.T., DeLuca, H.F., Vitamin D and multiple sclerosis. Proc Soc Exp Biol Med 216:121-27,1997

[25] Reynolds, E.H., Multiple sclerosis and vitamin B12 metabolism. J Neuroimmun 40:225-30,1992

[26] Ibid.

[27] Fischer, B.H., Marks, M. Reich, T., Hyperbaric-oxygen treatment of multiple sclerosis. A randomized, placebo-controlled, double-blind study. N Eng J Med 308(4):181-86,1983

[28] Barnes, M.P., Bates, D., Cartidge, N.E., Hyperbaric-oxygen and multiple sclerosis: final results of a placebo-controlled, double-blind trial. J Neurol Neurosurg Psychiatry 50(11):1402-6, 1987

[29] Davidson, D.L.W., Hyperbaric oxygen therapy in the treatment of multiple sclerosis: Report from Action for Research into Multiple Sclerosis, London, England, 1989

CHAPTER THREE

Amyotrophic Lateral Sclerosis

Amyotrophic Lateral Sclerosis (ALS) has been described as a "relentlessly progressive degenerative disorder" of the nervous system. Indeed, when reading medical texts and journals, the commentary dealing with this disorder is bleakly pessimistic.

ALS entered the public arena in the 1930's when Lou Gehrig, one of baseballs greatest players, was stricken with the disease. Gehrig earned the title "Iron Horse" for his record 2,130 consecutive games - a record ended by the debilitating effects of the disease that now bears his name.

About 1 or 2 of every 100,000 adult Americans are given the diagnosis of ALS each year and this incidence is increasing at an alarming rate.[1,2] Most commonly the disease is diagnosed between the ages of 55 and 75, but onset as early as the teenage years has been reported.[3] What typically follows is an exhaustive pursuit, often taking patients and their families to specialists practicing at the finest of the various "Clinics," only to leave hopelessly empty-handed.

The early symptoms of the disease are highly variable. Most commonly patients first experience weakness of an arm or leg. Other symptoms include difficulties with speech and swallowing, spasticity or stiffness of an extremity, difficulty controlling emotions, wasting of muscles, twitching of muscles (fasciculations) and shortness of breath.

With this diverse array of symptoms, misdiagnosis is always a concern. Many other neurological problems may mimic ALS to some degree and must therefore be judiciously excluded as diagnostic possibilities (see table 3.1).

Table 3.1 Diseases to exclude when diagnosing ALS

Parkinson's disease
post-polio syndrome
stroke
tumor of the base of the brain
spinal cord tumor
spinal cord cyst
multiple sclerosis
vitamin B12 deficiency
spinal stenosis (compromise of the spinal cord from
  overgrowth of bone)
peripheral neuropathy
myasthenia gravis
muscular dystrophy
inflammatory disease of muscle
Guillain Barré Syndrome

As of this writing, no specific "cure" for ALS has been identified. That is to say that no specific pharmaceutical company has as yet developed a patentable product that can be widely promoted to physicians for treating this disorder. The natural assumption that follows would be that medical researchers must not have much of an understanding of the mechanisms involved in causing ALS and allowing it to progress. But that is not the case. Virtually every team of scientists investigating ALS worldwide agree that the final common pathway mediating the destruction of brain neurons in ALS focuses on the central role of free radicals.[4] Excessive free radical activity in ALS seems to emanate from deficiencies of cellular energy production, a function normally carried out by the cell's power plant, the

The final common pathway mediating the destruction of brain neurons in ALS focuses on the central role of free radicals.

mitochondria. What likely compromises the effectiveness of the mitochondria to produce energy is an acquired or inherited genetic mutation as was elegantly described by British researchers in a recent publication.[5] Indeed, the free radical model coupled with defective neuronal energy production has become the dominant theme in all of the neurodegenerative diseases.[6]

Direct and powerful techniques for both protecting brain neurons from free radical damage as well as enhancing their energy production are widely described in our most highly regarded medical journals. Why then are patients and families told, "we're sorry, but nothing can be done"?

In November 1999 the American Academy of Neurology published a monograph defining the currently accepted approach to the treatment of ALS. In the entire text only one form of pharmaceutical intervention was described and it involved the use of a highly controversial medication, *riluzole*. While widely touted in medical journals as providing effective treatment for ALS patients, riluzole provides virtually no benefit and is associated with significant side effects in a large number of patients. As this most well respected journal reported, "It is often said that the benefits of riluzole are marginal but that side effects are major…The price of the drug is also often criticized, particularly if the patient's health care system does not pay for the drug. It is also of some concern that if the natural course of the disease and nature of the drug are not explained, the patient may develop false hopes. More generally, it is argued that the development of riluzole may retard the development of cheaper therapies because pharmaceutical companies and academic researchers may hesitate to invest in cheaper drugs, such as vitamin E…" And further, "Potential side effects also include psychological side effects, such as exaggerated hopes and secondary disappointment, which may interrupt the normal and beneficial coping process. Such problems are also most likely dependant on the attitude of the caregivers, and care must include providing complete information about the limits and opportunities of riluzole treatment."[7]

Aside from their comments on riluzole's lack of efficacy and side effect profile, the authors expose the real tragedy of ALS treatment. Potentially life saving approaches using powerful nonprescription antioxidants like vitamin E are ignored as they are "cheaper," that is to say, less profitable.

Clearly, riluzole does succeed at one important task. It allows treating physicians to end the day assured they "did something" for the ALS patients they are treating since a prescription was written – an obligation thus fulfilled.

Rational ALS Therapy

At the outset it must be stated that this protocol is not presented as a cure for amyotrophic lateral sclerosis. It is based upon the now well-described understanding of the fundamental biochemistry underlying this disorder and focuses on the two critical tasks of enhancing mitochondrial energetics and reducing free radical mediated neuronal damage. In addition, techniques designed to improve strength are incorporated into the protocol to enhance quality of life.

Cellular Energetics

Coenzyme Q10

Throughout this text we have explored the pivotal role of coenzyme Q10 in facilitating the fundamental processes of cellular energy production. Studies by Dr. M. Flynt Beal at the *Massachusetts General Hospital* confirm that this nutrient, taken by mouth, is readily absorbed, rapidly enters the bloodstream, and promotes a measurable improvement in mitochondrial energy production.[8] Unlike riluzole, coenzyme Q10 cannot be patented. This likely explains why no major pharmaceutical company is willing to step up to the plate and sponsor research to evaluate coenzyme Q10 for treating ALS. This is sad commentary, especially in light of the fact that coenzyme Q10 dramatically extends survival in animal models of ALS.[9] So there is no reason to wait for clinical research to prove coenzyme Q10's effectiveness in humans. Time is clearly of the essence in ALS. Including coenzyme Q10 in this protocol is mandatory.

Coenzyme Q10 dramatically extends survival in animal models of ALS.

Acetyl-L-Carnitine

Like coenzyme Q10, acetyl-L-carnitine functions as a critical player in the process by which neurons create energy. Its role is twofold. First, acetyl-L-carnitine acts as a carrier of fatty acids, delivering them to the mitochondria where they serve as fuels for energy production. Maintaining adequate mitochondrial function requires efficient elimination of metabolic waste products, and this is acetyl-L-carnitine's second task.

Phosphatidylserine

Within the mitochondria, energy is produced in a highly convoluted structure known as the mitochondrial membrane. The ability of the mitochondrial membrane to function adequately requires not only an adequate supply of fuel and important cofactors like niacin, pyridoxine and coenzyme Q10, but also one very important structural component, phosphatidylserine. Its ability to enhance brain performance has not yet been evaluated in ALS, but its striking benefit in Alzheimer's disease supports its inclusion in this protocol.[10]

Antioxidant Protection

Glutathione

Glutathione represents one of the most critical and powerful antioxidants protecting delicate neurons from the ravages of free radical induced damage. As such, it is the subject of intense medical research being described in more than 40,000 articles listed in the *Medline* database.

Intriguing research published in 1999 by Japanese scientists has revealed a striking deficiency of this brain-protecting chemical in the cerebrospinal fluid of patients diagnosed with amyotrophic lateral sclerosis.[11] As the now widely accepted model of ALS recognizes the pivotal role of free radicals as the causative agent in neuronal damage, this report, showing deficiency of glutathione in ALS patients, has profound implications. Not only may glutathione deficiency play a role in the genesis of ALS, but its repletion offers the potential for a powerful therapeutic intervention. Glutathione's potential for treating ALS is supported by recently published research from *Harvard Medical School*. The authors stated, " Pertubations of free radical homeostasis are proposed to cause ALS. A corollary hypothesis is that antioxidants should slow the disease course. One strategy for antioxidant therapy is to manipulate levels of glutathione…" This report, published in the April 1999 issue of the journal *Neurology*, demonstrated that a proprietary product, *Procysteine*, was able to increase brain levels of glutathione. Obviously its manufacturer recognizes glutathione's potential as an ALS treatment. This explains why at the conclusion of the paper it is disclosed that they provided financial support for the study.[12]

There's one more important reason why glutathione is included in the BrainRecovery.com protocol. Epidemiological studies have long confirmed a substantial increased risk of developing ALS in individuals with a history of occupational exposure to agricultural chemicals.[13] But the percentage of exposed individuals who go on to develop

ALS is obviously quite small. What then is unique about this small number of people who ultimately develop ALS following this form of toxic exposure? Clearly, the answer lies in how their bodies respond to the toxic insult. That is to say that some individuals may be at increased risk for developing ALS following exposure to a toxin because of inadequacies of their detoxification systems. This thesis has been validated by extensive research that clearly confirms the fact that abnormalities of liver detoxification activity are frequently observed in ALS patients.[14]

The effectiveness of an individual's detoxification ability is readily assessed by performing a *Hepatic Detoxifiction Profile*, available from Great Smokies Diagnostic Laboratory (see below). This test not only demonstrates specific detoxification abnormalities, but also provides suggestions for specific therapeutic interventions.

One of the most critical components of hepatic detoxification is glutathione. Glutathione deficiency is directly linked to reduced effectiveness of the detoxification process. This adds further support for the inclusion of glutathione in this protocol.

Glutathione is not effective when given orally. The BrainRecovery.com protocol therefore incorporates intravenous injection of this naturally occurring antioxidant. Its administration is simple, and it is inexpensive and well tolerated (see below).

In addition to providing glutathione intravenously, specific oral nutritional supplements can greatly enhance the body's ability to produce glutathione, thus offering further antioxidant protection. N-acetyl-cysteine (NAC) is such a supplement. Widely available in health food stores, NAC not only increases glutathione, but serves as a powerful antioxidant in and of itself. It has potent efficacy in

Abnormalities of liver detoxification activity are frequently observed in ALS patients.

reducing the activity of the powerful free radical, *nitric oxide*.[15] This is a particularly timely discovery, since the latest research reveals that nitric oxide production in ALS patients may be as much as 73% increased compared to controls.[16]

Vitamin E

The high fat content of brain tissue makes fat-soluble vitamin E an ideal candidate as a therapeutic antioxidant in neurodegenerative conditions. This explains why it is currently the focus of extensive study in the treatment of Parkinson's disease, multiple sclerosis, Alzheimer's disease, as well as ALS. Deficiency of this important brain protecting antioxidant creates an environment more favorable for free radical damage of delicate brain and spinal cord tissue. In fact, brain levels of vitamin E in ALS patients may be as much as 31% lower than normal.[17]

Vitamin E both delayed the onset and slowed the progression of ALS in mice with a genetic form of the disease.

Researchers at *Northwestern University Medical School* have now concluded that vitamin E both delayed the onset and slowed the progression of ALS in mice with a genetic form of the disease. Although there was no prolongation of survival, these experimental animals showed preservation of function for a longer period of time.[18] This has obvious implications in humans in terms of quality of life.

Vitamin D

It is now clear that vitamin D is far more important in human physiology than simply aiding in bone formation and maintenance. Its deficiency has been noted in multiple sclerosis, Parkinson's disease, and now ALS as well.[19,20,21] Incredibly, the conclusion reached by the researchers discovering this deficiency was simply that these patients were at increased risk for bone fractures related to osteoporosis. Exploring the vast array of biological activities of vitamin D in the human would have led these scientists to the understanding that vitamin D has profound antioxidant activity – rivaling vitamin E, and that the deficiency of this fat-soluble antioxidant may play an important *causative* role in these and other neurodegenerative conditions.[22] Their conclusions should have focused on vitamin D's therapeutic potential for these challenging brain disorders.

Alpha Lipoic Acid

Alpha lipoic acid is clearly the most exciting antioxidant of the decade. And rightfully so. Unlike more familiar antioxidants, alpha lipoic acid is not categorized as being "water soluble" or "fat soluble." It is both.[23] This has profound implications in terms of its absorption from the gut as it is able gain access to the body using pathways for both fat and water soluble nutrients. Its fat solubility provides another benefit – it facilitates the ability of this powerful antioxidant to enter the brain. This makes it an ideal candidate for the neurodegenerative conditions.

The antioxidant activity of alpha lipoic acid may be more powerful than that of vitamin E. But even more important, it has the unique ability to regenerate many of the other vital brain antioxidants including vitamins E, C, and glutathione.[24]

Finally, alpha lipoic acid acts as a metal chelator, binding potentially dangerous free radical inducing chemicals like cadmium, iron, copper, and zinc.[25]

Vitamin C

Also an important brain antioxidant, vitamin C serves to support the activity of other brain antioxidants including vitamin E, glutathione, and lipoic acid. Its importance in ALS is supported by the observation that a commonly used animal model for ALS research is a genetically unique guinea pig – unique in that it does not produce vitamin C.[26] This may explain why the *Linus Pauling Institute* uses high dosage vitamin C in their protocol for ALS.[27]

Ginkgo biloba

With the exciting publication in the *Journal of the American Medical Association* revealing the effectiveness of Ginkgo biloba in treating Alzheimer's disease, researchers are now exploring the use of this ancient herb in the treatment of other neurodegenerative diseases.[28] And with good reason. Not only does Ginkgo biloba posses significant brain antioxidant activity, but it also enhances brain blood flow and neuronal metabolism.[29]

Improving Strength

Creatine

In a recent report appearing in the journal *Neurology*, Canadian researchers demonstrated a marked increase in several parameters of strength in subjects consuming high doses of the oral supplement creatine. None of the subjects suffered from ALS, but a variety of other neurodegenerative conditions were described. Patients diagnosed with post-polio syndrome experienced a significant benefit from the treatment and this is relevant since the specific neurons which degenerate in this syndrome are the same ones destroyed in ALS. The dosages used in the study ranged from 5-10 grams daily. Further, this study and others have failed to identify any significant side effects.[30]

But there's even more exciting news supporting creatine supplementation for ALS patients. Researchers at *Harvard Medical School* have been hard at work looking for ways to both protect brain neurons and improve motor performance in mice with a genetic form of ALS in hopes of uncovering some form of intervention that could benefit ALS patients. In March 1999 they published truly impressive results revealing that creatine

"Creatine administration may be a new therapeutic strategy for ALS."

supplementation accomplishes both tasks. Creatine was found to produce a "...dose-dependant improvement in motor performance and extended survival..." The authors concluded, "Therefore, creatine administration may be a new therapeutic strategy for ALS."[31]

These studies provide substantial support for the inclusion of creatine in the **BrainRecovery.com** protocol for ALS. It is unfortunate that for the simple fact that a nutritional supplement like creatine is not a prescription item, its potential goes unnoticed, despite supportive research from our most highly regarded institutions.

Human Growth Hormone

As with the use of creatine described above, our incorporation of human growth hormone in the treatment protocol for ALS patients is a natural extension of the positive results we have observed in patients with post-polio syndrome. Almost uniformly, ALS patients gain an improved sense of well-being after beginning growth hormone injections.

Many researchers have looked upon ALS as simply representing a manifestation of accelerated aging of a specific part of the nervous system. Human growth hormone has been shown to have a positive effect on a number of aging parameters including: lowering blood pressure, improving kidney function, increasing energy level, enhancing sexual performance, increasing cardiac output, increasing bone strength, enhancing wound healing, improving vision, increasing memory retention, and improving sleep.[32] These findings justify the inclusion of human growth hormone administration in the **BrainRecovery.com** protocol for ALS.

BrainRecovery.com
ALS Protocol

Intravenous Glutathione

Our protocol for using glutathione is relatively simple. Glutathione is inexpensive and easily obtained (see below). We use liquid glutathione, not reconstituted powder. It should be administered, at least initially, by a qualified healthcare practitioner as follows:

1. Dilute the appropriate dosage of glutathione liquid in 10 cc of sterile normal saline. Usually vials contain 200mg, but read the label.
2. This solution is then injected through a 21-gauge butterfly catheter intravenously over a 15 to 20 minute period of time.
3. Alternatively, many patients choose to have intravenous access ports inserted. This allows frequent glutathione administration without repeated needle sticks.
4. Treatment begins at 600mg glutathione 3 times a week and may be increased to daily injections of up to 800mg depending on results. Alternatively, a schedule of 1400mg glutathione 3 times a week may be utilized.

A complete instructional video for glutathione administration is available by calling *i*Nutritionals, at: (800) 530-1982, or may be ordered by visiting www.BrainRecovery.com

Injectable glutathione is available from:

> Wellness Health and Pharmaceuticals
> 2800 South 18th Street
> Birmingham, Alabama 35209
> Tel. (800) 227-2627
> Fax. (800) 369-0302

Their web site can be accessed by visiting:
www.BrainRecovery.com

Human Growth Hormone

Human growth hormone (Humatrope®) is given by intramuscular injection - 2mg, 3 times each week. This dosage, based on a 70 kg adult, is slowly increased over 2-3 months to 4mg, 3 times a week. Patients should be told to watch for side effects such as ankle swelling, tingling or numbness in the first 3 fingers (carpal tunnel syndrome), or breast enlargement. These experiences are fortunately quite rare. We have found that our patients easily learn how to self-administer this medication, a technique easily learned from the treating physician or nurse.

Because of the potential for abuse of human growth hormone by individuals seeking to improve their athletic performance, some pharmacies will not accept prescriptions from any physician except an endocrinologist. This may require ordering the drug from a compounding pharmacy.

A list of physicians using human growth hormone can be found in the book, *Grow Young with HGH*, (see resources section below).

Vitamins and Antioxidants

	daily dose
Vitamin B3	100 mg
Vitamin B6	100 mg
Vitamin C	2500 - 3000 mg
Vitamin E	2400 IU
Alpha lipoic acid	80 mg
N-Acetyl Cysteine	400 mg
Ginkgo Biloba	60 mg
Vitamin D	400 IU

Cellular Energizers

	daily dose
Coenzyme Q10	200-300 mg
Phosphatidylserine	100 mg
Acetyl-L-carnitine	400 mg
Creatine	6-8 gms

Or, if using the Brain Sustain™ supplement:

Glutathione and human growth hormone as above, and:

Brain Sustain™ _____ 2 scoops daily

Vitamin C_____ 2000 mg daily

Vitamin E _____ 2000 IU daily

Coenzyme Q10_____ 140-240 mg daily

Creatine _____ 6-8 gms daily

Note :

Because Liver detoxification abnormalities are so prevalent in ALS, perform a *Hepatic Detoxification Profile*
available from:

> Great Smokies Diagnostic Laboratory
> 63 Zillicoa Street
> Asheville, N.C. 28801-9801
> Tel. (800) 522 – 4762

If hepatic detoxification abnormalities are detected :

1. MediClear® _____ Week 1: 1 scoop twice daily
    _____ Week 2: 1 scoop three times each day
    _____ Week 3: 1 scoop three times each day
    _____ Week 4: 1 scoop one time daily
2. Silymarin _____ 200 mg - twice daily

3. Intravenous glutathione as described above

After 4 weeks discontinue MediClear®, continue silymarin , and intravenous glutathione and begin the standard BrainRecovery.com ALS Protocol described above.

MediClear® must be ordered by a *licensed health-care practitioner* and is available from:

> Thorne Research, Inc.
> 25820 Highway 2 West
> PO Box 25
> Dover, Idaho 83825
> Tel. (800) 228-1966

Resources

1. Grow Young with HGH, by Dr. Robert Klatz. HarperCollins, New York, ISBN 0-06-018682-8, 1997
2. Les Turner Amyotrophic Lateral Sclerosis Foundation 8142 Lawndale Ave. Skokie, Il 60076 Phone: (847) 679-3311 Web Site: www.lesturnerals.org

BrainSustain is a nutritional supplement designed to maintain health brain function. It is not intended to treat or cure any

References

[1] Kurtzke, J.K., Risk factors in amyotrophic lateral sclerosis. In Rowland, L.P., (ed): Amyotrophic Lateral Sclerosis and Other Motor Neuron Diseases, 245-270, New York, Raven Press, 1991

[2] Brooks, B.R., Clinical epidemiology of ALS, in Riggs J.E., (ed), Neurology Clinics; 14:399-420, Philadelphia, W.B. Saunders, 1991

[3] Ibid

[4] Gutmann, L., and Mitsumoto, H., Advances in ALS, Neurology; 47 (Suppl 2): S17-18, 1999

[5] Borthwick, G. M., Johnson, M.A., Ince, P.G., et al., Mitochondrial Enzyme Activity In Amyotrophic Lateral Sclerosis: Implications for the Role of Mitochondria in Cell Death. Ann Neurol 46: 787-790, 1999

[6] Beal, M.F., Hyman, B.T., and Koroshetz, W., Do defects in mitochondrial energy metabolism underlie the pathology of neurodegenerative disease? Trends Neurosci; 16:125-131, 1993

[7] Ludolph, A.C., and Riepe, M.W., Do the benefits of currently available treatments justify early diagnosis and treatment of amyotrophic lateral sclerosis? Arguments against. Neurology 53 (Suppl 5): S46-S49, 1999

[8] Shults, C.W., Beal, M.F., Fontaine, K. et al., Absorption, tolerability and effects on mitochondrial activity of oral coenzyme Q10 in parkinsonian patients, Neurology 50: 793-795,1998

[9] Beal, M.F., Coenzyme Q10 administration and its potential for treatment of neurodegenerative diseases. Biofactors 9 (2-4): 261-6, 1999

[10] Crook, T.H., Tinklenberg, J., Yesavage, J., Effects of phosphatidylserine in age-associated memory impairment. Neurology 41:644-49, 1991

[11] Tohgi, H., Abe, T., Yamazaki, K., et al., Increase in oxidized NO products and reduction in oxidized glutathione in cerebrospinal fluid from patients with sporadic form of amyotrophic lateral sclerosis. Neurosci Lett 260(3):204-6, 1999

[12] Cudkowitz, M.E., Sexton, B.S., Ellis, B.A., et al., The pharmacokinetics and pharmacodynamics of Procysteine in amyotrophic lateral sclerosis. Neurology 52: 1492-1494, 1999

[13] Baker, B., ALS Tied to Agricultural Chemical Exposure at Work: Strongest Link in Men Exposed Under Age 40. Family Practice News: pp.1,2, May 15, 1996

[14] Steventon, G., Williams, A.C., Waring, R.H., et al., Xenobiotic metabolism in motor neuron disease. Lancet 2 (8612): 644-7, 1988

[15] Pahan, K., Sheikh, G.S., Nmboodiri, A.M.S., et al., N-acetyl cysteine inhibits induction of NO production by endotoxin or cytokine stimulated rat peritoneal macrophages, C6 glial cells and astrocytes. Free Radical Biology and Medicine 24(1):39-48, 1998

[16] Tohgi, H., Abe, T., Yamazaki, K., et al., Increase in oxidized NO products and reduction in oxidized glutathione in cerebrospinal fluid from patients with sporadic form of amyotrophic lateral sclerosis. Neurosci Lett 260(3):204-6, 1999

[17] Hideo, H., et al., α-Tocopherol Quinine Level is Remarkably Low in the Cerebrospinal Fluid of Patients with Sporadic Amyotrophic Lateral Sclerosis. Neurosciences Letter 207: 5-8, 1996

[18] Gurney, M.E., Cutting, F.B., Zhai, P., et al., Benefit of vitamin E, riluzole, and gabapentin in a transgenic model of familial amyotrophic lateral sclerosis. Ann Neurol 39(2): 147-57, 1996

[19] Nieves, J., Cosman, F., Shen, H.J. et al., High prevalence of vitamin D deficiency and reduced bone mass in multiple sclerosis. Neurology 44(9): 1687-92, 1994

[20] Sato, Y., Kikuyama, M., Oizumi, K., High prevalence of vitamin D deficiency and reduced bone mass in Parkinson's disease. Neurology 49(5): 1273-78, 1997

[21] Sato. Y., Honda, Y., Asoh, T., et al., Hypovitaminosis D and decreased bone mineral density in amyotrophic lateral sclerosis. Eur Neurol 37(4): 225-9, 1997

[22] Sardar, S., Chakraborty, A., and Chatterjee, M., Comparative effectiveness of vitamin D3 and dietary vitamin E on peroxidation of lipids and enzymes of the hepatic antioxidant system in Sprague – Dawley rats. Int J Vitam Nutr Res, 66(1): 39-45, 1996

[23] Marangon, K., Devaraj, S., Tirosh, O., et al., Comparison of the effect of α-lipoic acid and α-tocopherol supplementation on measures of oxidative stress. Free Radical Biology & Medicine 27(9/10): 1114-1121, 1999

[24] Ibid

[25] Ibid

[26] Kok, A.B., Ascorbate availability and neurodegeneration in amyotrophic lateral sclerosis

[27] Ringrose, C.A., Therapeutic use of IV vitamin C in degenerative diseases. The Linus Pauling Institute of Science and Medicine Newsletter (8) ,1994

[28] Le Bars, P., Katz, M.M., Berman, N., et al., A Placebo-Controlled, Double-blind Randomized Trial of an Extract of Ginkgo Biloba for Dementia. JAMA 278(16):1327-32,1997

[29] Ibid

[30] Tarnopolsky, M., Martin, J., Creatine monohydrate increases strength in patients with neuromuscular disease. Neurology 52: 854-57, 1999

[31] Klivenyi, P., Ferrante, R.J., Mathews R.T., et al., Neuroprotective effects of creatine in a transgenic animal model of amyotrophic lateral sclerosis. Nat Med 5(3): 347-50, 1999

[32] Klatz, R., *Grow Young with HGH*. New York: HarperCollins, 1997, p. 9

CHAPTER FOUR

Post-Polio Syndrome

Poliomyelitis, now a rarity in the United States, is a viral induced illness which reached epidemic levels in the United States in the late 1940's to the mid 1950's. Fortunately, an effective vaccination program led to a dramatic decline in new cases. While new cases are exceedingly rare, there are nevertheless an estimated 300,000 polio survivors in the United States today - 25% of whom experience symptoms of so called "post-polio syndrome."[1]

Post-polio syndrome is an illness in which polio survivors experience weakness in muscles previously affected by the initial polio infection. The onset of post-polio syndrome may occur any time between 10 and 40 years after recovery from the initial polio event. There is a direct relationship between the severity of post-polio syndrome and the severity of the initial polio infection. Typically, individuals who had only minor muscle weakness with their original polio infection as a rule experience only mild symptoms of post-polio syndrome. In others, often those who experienced severe weakness originally, post-polio syndrome can cause profound muscle weakness with feelings of generalized fatigue, joint and muscle pain, and continued loss of muscle bulk.[2]

The cause of post-polio syndrome has not yet been fully elucidated. It is certainly well known that a specific virus causes the original polio infection and there has been some speculation that post-polio syndrome may represent some form of reactivation of this latent virus. But as yet, this has not been fully demonstrated.

Another theory relates post-polio syndrome to the normal process of nervous system aging. This theory holds that all parts of the nervous system age at a fairly constant rate which continues throughout an individual's lifetime. The original polio infection may simply have advanced this aging process by a quantum leap.

The diagnosis of post-polio syndrome is typically made based upon a full understanding of a patient's history, with particular emphasis on understanding the initial event of polio, and the physical examination. It may at times be confused with other diseases characterized by progressive weakness as seen in table 4.1. This is why various ancillary studies are often part of the evaluation. These tests include magnetic resonance imaging (MRI) studies of the spine and brain, spinal fluid analysis (lumbar puncture), electromyography (EMG), and nerve conduction studies. These are tests designed to exclude other conditions since there is as yet no specific definitive test available to diagnose post-polio syndrome. There has been no isolation of any virus felt to be causative in this illness, nor is there any evidence that this condition is in any way contagious.

There has been no isolation of any virus felt to be causative in this illness.

Until recently, attempts at treating post-polio syndrome have been disappointing. Studies at the *National Institutes of Health* (NIH) have evaluated treating post-polio patients with the immune regulating chemical *interferon*, but this has proven ineffective. Steroids have been tried and these studies have likewise demonstrated no improvement. Other drugs, which have been evaluated and proven essentially useless, include *pyridostigmine* and *amantadine*.[3]

But one area of research that clearly shows promise is the use of so called "growth factors" which are substances known to increase the branching of nerve terminals and enhance the way nerves provide information to muscles. Soon, a multi-center trial will begin to evaluate insulin-like growth factor (IGF-1) in the treatment of post-polio syndrome. But while the use of IGF-1 in post-polio syndrome seems promising, it is still very much in the experimental stage.[4]

Table 4.1 .	Diseases to exclude when diagnosing post-polio syndrome

brachial neuritis (inflammation of the nerves of the upper extremity)
amyotrophic lateral sclerosis
tumor of the base of the brain
spinal cord tumor
spinal cord cyst
multiple sclerosis
vitamin B12 deficiency
spinal stenosis (compromise of the spinal cord from overgrowth of bone)
peripheral neuropathy
myasthenia gravis
muscular dystrophy
inflammatory disease of muscle
Guillain Barré Syndrome

If post-polio syndrome does indeed represent simply an advanced form of aging of the nervous system, then it would make sense to at least take a look at any pharmaceutical agent that could conceivably slow down parameters of this process. There is a medicine that can do just that, and its called *human growth hormone*. Human growth hormone has been popularized as of late as a so-called "fountain of youth drug" - a title that is somewhat justifiable. In the book "Grow Young with HGH" (human growth hormone), author Dr. Ronald Klatz summarizes the various studies of human growth hormone documenting its effect in a number of measures of aging including its ability to lower blood pressure, improve kidney function, increase energy level, enhance sexual performance, increase cardiac output, enhance immune functions, improve cholesterol profile with higher HDL and lower LDL, increase bone strength, enhance wound healing, sharpen vision, increase memory retention, and improve sleep.[5] Indeed human growth hormone has become one of the cornerstones of treatment in various anti-aging clinics.

In early 1998, we began administering human growth hormone to patients with post-polio syndrome. The results have been nothing short of dramatic. Typically patients who have been experiencing progressive decline in muscle function have experienced not only stabilization, but also actual *improvement* of muscle strength. Here are reports from two of our patients suffering from post-polio syndrome who are now using human growth hormone:

T.N. is a 65 year-old-gentleman who sustained a fairly advanced case of poliomyelitis at age 22 years. He was hospitalized for 4 months spending most of that time in an "iron lung." He was then on crutches for 3 years. Thereafter, he was never able to run or go up steps without at least some difficulty and had been left with some fairly severe weakness of the left leg. As he stated:

> "I was steadily losing strength and had other problems until I started growth hormone injections nine months ago. My overall strength has improved for the first time in thirteen years. One thing I notice most is the ability to get up from a chair without difficulty. Before growth hormone I would sometimes have to make more than one attempt to raise to standing.
>
> The second benefit is my stamina has increased to the point that I can get through a large airport without resting several times.
>
> Lastly, my sleep (I have sleep apnea) has improved more than any time in forty years."

Here's another report describing the effectiveness of human growth hormone from a 60 year old retired engineer:

Dear Dr. Perlmutter,

I am a 60 year old male who had polio at the age of 5 that affected primarily the muscles in my legs (quadriceps) and lower back. In my teenage years, due to a regimen of exercise and weight training, I maintained good mobility and strength and was able to participate in most activities normal to teenagers. When entering the early 40's, I began to experience a great deal of leg pain and the muscles in my legs had begun to weaken. By the time I was in my late 40's, the weakness and pain became so significant, I went through a series of tests at Henry Ford Hospital in Michigan. It was then that I was diagnosed with post-polio syndrome. At 50 years of age, I fully retired and moved to Florida. Although I continued with a regimen of exercise, healthy diet, and vitamin supplements, I noticed that my legs had grown progressively weaker. By the time I turned 60, in addition to the leg weakness I also began to experience muscle wasting in my arms. Up to this point in my life, I always had good upper body strength and muscles due to the weight training, so I became very concerned and started to do a great deal of research to try to find a possible solution to this problem. A few months ago, I read an article by Dr. Perlmutter describing the work he was doing with patients suffering from post-polio syndrome. After an extensive examination and interview, Dr. Perlmutter started me on a program using human growth hormone and nutritional supplements. After only 6 weeks using the human growth the results have been startling. By the 4th week, the muscle wasting in my arms has reversed to the point that they are as good as they were when I was 40. Before starting the treatment I could barely walk to the mailbox in front of my house. Now, I can easily walk a mile.

I thought my life would end short, but now I'm looking forward to better years.

Your most grateful patient,

H.C.

Human growth hormone administration

Human growth hormone (Humatrope®) is given by intramuscular injection - 2mg, 3 times each week. This dosage, based on a 70 kg adult, is slowly increased over 2-3 months to 4mg, 3 times a week. Patients should be told to watch for side effects such as ankle swelling, tingling or numbness in the first 3 fingers (carpal tunnel syndrome), or breast enlargement. These experiences are fortunately quite rare. We have found that our patients easily learn how to self-administer this medication, a technique easily learned from the treating physician or nurse.

Because of the potential for abuse of human growth hormone by individuals seeking to improve their athletic performance, some pharmacies will not accept prescriptions from any physician except an endocrinologist. This may require ordering the drug from a compounding pharmacy (see below).

Cellular Energetics

Enhancing the metabolic activity of damaged but functional neurons is a primary goal in the treatment of post-polio syndrome. This can be accomplished with the following nutrients:

Creatine

Visit any popular gym or fitness club and you're likely to find that *creatine monohydrate* is one of their best selling nutritional supplements. And with good reason. Studies have long demonstrated convincing evidence of the benefit of creatine supplementation in several indices of athletic performance.

Because of creatine's benefit in athletes, researchers have studied its possible role in various neurological disorders. In a 1999 study published in the journal *Neurology*, Canadian researchers tested the effectiveness of creatine monohydrate in post-polio syndrome as well as several other conditions characterized by muscle weakness. The results were impressive. There was an increase in both upper and lower extremity strength, with an actual increase in muscle mass not only in the patients with post-polio syndrome, but in several other conditions as well including, muscular dystrophy, inflammatory muscle disease, and neuropathy.[6]

The study was short term – only 10 days, but our experience with long term usage of creatine demonstrates continued benefit and safety of this nutritional supplement. Typical adult dosage is 6-8 grams of creatine monohydrate each day. Individuals consuming a diet high in meat may find beneficial results from a lower dosage, in the 4-5 gram per day range.

Acetyl-L-carnitine

Acting in many ways similar to creatine, acetyl-L-carnitine enhances the metabolic activity of neurons by serving as a transporter of metabolic fuels to the energy producing machinery of the cell, the mitochondria. Aside from bringing the "coal to the furnace," acetyl-L-carnitine further aids in energy production by assisting in the removal of toxic by-products of metabolism.

Coenzyme Q10   (CoQ10)

Essential for the viability of everything living, CoQ10 is an enzyme which facilitates the fundamental biochemical processes involved in cellular energy production. Since abnormalities of muscle cell metabolism are at the heart of post-polio syndrome, CoQ10 is receiving a lot of attention as an adjunct to the treatment of this disease.

Danish researchers using highly sophisticated techniques to evaluate muscle cell metabolism have now demonstrated significant improvements in muscle cell energy production in the calf muscle of post-polio syndrome patients following CoQ10 administration. The researchers invoked three mechanisms for the beneficial action of CoQ10 including: improvement in blood circulation to the affected muscles, enhanced cellular energy production, and a reduction in free radical activity.[7]

Danish researchers have now demonstrated significant improvements in muscle cell energy production in the calf muscle of post-polio syndrome patients following CoQ10 administration.

Nicotinamide Adenine Dinucleotide (NADH)

Like CoQ10, NADH is a critical enzyme in the biochemical pathway for energy production. Having demonstrated its effectiveness in various other neurodegenerative disorders like Alzheimer's disease, Parkinson's disease, as well as chronic fatigue syndrome, the energy enhancing potential of NADH secures its inclusion in the BrainRecovery.com protocol for post-polio syndrome.

Antioxidant Protection

Whether post-polio syndrome represents an accelerated aging phenomenon or a reactivation of a latent virus, the final common pathway destroying the neurons is mediated by *free radicals*. Free radicals are destructive chemicals normally found in all living systems; formed during the process of energy metabolism. It is the progressive destruction of the body's tissues and DNA by free radical activity that is responsible for the process we call aging. Normally, our bodies successfully quench these potentially damaging free radicals almost instantaneously after they are formed. This is the job of the various *antioxidants* that we produce and consume. Obviously it makes sense to enhance antioxidant potential in post-polio syndrome, and in any other degenerative condition for that matter.

Alpha-Lipoic Acid

The discovery of the antioxidant potential of alpha lipoic acid will rank as one of the most important advances in the treatment of neurodegenerative diseases this decade. Its usefulness in protecting the nervous system from damaging free radicals has been the subject of extensive research. Why lipoic acid has attracted so much attention centers upon at least three unique characteristics. First, more than almost any other antioxidant, lipoic acid readily crosses the blood-brain barrier becoming available to the entire central nervous system. Second, lipoic acid actually enhances the regeneration of other antioxidants in the brain including vitamins C and E, and glutathione. Finally, lipoic acid acts as a metal chelator. That means it binds and enhances the excretion of various potentially toxic metals, which may otherwise encourage the production of free radicals.

Lipoic acid readily crosses the blood-brain barrier becoming available to the entire central nervous system.

Vitamin E

Perhaps the most popular antioxidant worldwide, vitamin E should be included in the post-polio program since it is one of the main antioxidants of the nervous system. Being a fat-soluble antioxidant, vitamin E helps reduce free radicals in fat-containing tissues like the brain and peripheral nerves. Its ability to quench free radicals in the brain likely explains its profound effectiveness in slowing the progression of Alzheimer's disease and why it is advocated in Parkinson's disease as well. With many vitamins, there is very little difference in quality between discounted brands and more expensive labels. Not so with vitamin E. Supermarkets and drugstores frequently carry low quality and inexpensive vitamin E products. Read the fine print. The vitamin E to choose is *d-alpha tocopherol*. Avoid the synthetic *dl-alpha tocopherol*. It may seem like a small distinction, but there is a profound difference in the biological activities of these two products. Also, vitamin E, being oil based, should be refrigerated to preserve its potency.

Glutathione

Also an important brain antioxidant, glutathione has been the subject of intense study as of late because of its critical role in brain aging. Like alpha lipoic acid, glutathione helps to recycle vitamins C and E, and may also enhance the activity of *neurotransmitters*. These are the chemical messengers allowing neurons the ability to communicate with each other. Unfortunately, glutathione cannot itself be given orally since it is rapidly digested to its constituent amino acids. This explains why we administer glutathione intravenously as part of our protocol in the treatment of Parkinson's disease, and why I.V. glutathione may become a part of our protocol for post-polio syndrome in the future. Fortunately, there is a nutritional supplement which has been found to significantly enhance the body's natural production of glutathione. It is the modified amino acid *N-acetyl cysteine* or NAC, which in addition to encouraging glutathione production, possesses antioxidant properties in its own right.

Vitamin C

This vitamin also falls into the category of "brain antioxidants." It works in concert with vitamin E, lipoic acid and glutathione. It's important to emphasize that the main antioxidants in the brain, vitamins C and E, glutathione, and alpha lipoic acid all work in concert, protecting against the damaging effect of free radicals in slightly different ways. Deficiencies of one or more of these agents creates a weak link in the chain, paving the way for an increased damage from free radical activity.

Vitamin D

Like vitamin E, this important antioxidant is fat soluble making it an ideal candidate for neurological conditions. Recent research shows that the antioxidant activity of vitamin D may actually exceed that of vitamin E. We are only now just beginning to recognize that vitamin D has many important roles in human physiology aside from helping to maintain bone density.

BrainRecovery.com
Post-Polio Syndrome Protocol

Human Growth Hormone (Humatrope®) Dosage for a 70 kg adult: 2mg IM, 3 days each week increasing to 4mg IM, 3 days weekly after 2 months. Injectable Human Growth Hormone can be obtained from:

> Wellness Health and Pharmaceuticals
> 2800   South 18th Street
> Birmingham, Alabama 35209
> Tel. (800) 227-2627
> Fax. (800) 369-0302

Their web site can be accessed by visiting:
www.BrainRecovery.com

A list of physicians using human growth hormone can be found in the book, *Grow Young with HGH*, (see resources section).

Antioxidants

	daily dose
Alpha Lipoic Acid	80 mg
N-acetyl Cysteine	400 mg
Vitamin E	1200 IU
Vitamin C	800 mg
Ginkgo biloba	60 mg
Vitamin D	400 IU

Cellular Energizers

Coenzyme Q10	60 mg
Creatine monohydrate	4-6 grams
Acetyl-L-carnitine	400 mg
NADH	5mg twice daily

Or, if using the **Brain Sustain**™ supplement:

Human growth hormone, NADH and creatine monohydrate as above, and :

Brain Sustain™ _____ 2 scoops daily

Vitamin E _____ 800 units daily

BrainSustain is a nutritional supplement designed to maintain healthy brain function. It is not intended to treat or cure any specific disease.

Resources

1. Post-Polio syndrome. Edited by Lauro S. Halstead and Gunnar Grimby. Hanley & Belfus, Philadelphia, 1995.
2. A Summer Plague: polio and Its Survivors. Tony Gould. Yale University Press, 1995.
3. Current Trends in Post-Poliomyelitis Syndrome. Daria A. Trojan and Neil R. Cashman.Milestone Medical Communications, New York. 1996.
4. Post-Polio Syndrome: A New Challenge for the Survivors of Polio. A CD-ROM Published by Bioscience Communications, New York.
5. Managing Post-Polio: A Guide To Living Well With Post-Polio Syndrome: Edited by Lauro S. Halstead. NRH Press and ABI Professional Publications, Falls Church, Va., 1998.
6. Grow Young with HGH, by Dr. Robert Klatz. HarperCollins, New York, ISBN 0-06-018682-8, 1997

References

[1] Post-polio fact sheet, NIH Publication No. 96-4030, National Institutes of Health, 1996

[2] Ibid.

[3] Ibid

[4] Ibid

[5] Klatz, R., *Grow Young with HGH*. New York: HarperCollins, 1997, p. 9

[6] Tarnopolsky, M., Martin, J., Creatine monohydrate increases strength in patients with neuromuscular disease. Neurology 52: 854-57, 1999

[7] Mizuno, M., Quistorff, B., Theorell, H., et al., Effects of oral supplementation of coenzyme Q10 on 31P-NMR detected skeletal muscle energy metabolism in middle-aged post-polio subjects and normal volunteers. Mol Aspects Med 18 (Suppl.): S291-98

CHAPTER FIVE

Alzheimer's Disease

As the 20th century comes to a close, we are witnessing a staggering increase in dementing illnesses. At present, approximately 4.5 million Americans have Alzheimer's disease. By the year 2030, it has been estimated that this number will approach 9 million. Prevalence of Alzheimer's disease has been estimated to be 50 % in individuals 85 years or older – the most rapidly growing segment of our population (see figure 5.1). Estimates of annual costs for the care of these patients approach $60 billion in the U.S. alone.[1] Any effective treatment that could delay the onset of Alzheimer's by just 5 years would reduce the cost to society by as much as $30 billion annually.[2] But the emotional costs borne by families and caregivers are immeasurable.

In our magic-bullet society where physicians and patients alike are programmed to turn to the pharmaceutical industry to cure our ills, it appears that we have come up empty-handed when confronted by dementia. Nevertheless, our medical journals continue to display large compelling advertisements extolling the effectiveness of various so called "Alzheimer's drugs." But in a recent issue of *Archives of Neurology* (June 1999,) the lack of usefulness of any of these drugs was eloquently described in a guest editorial by Dr. William Pryse-Phillips.[3]

Prevalence of Alzheimer's disease has been estimated to be 50 % in individuals 85 years or older.

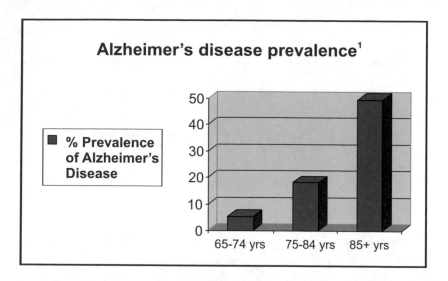

Figure 5.1. Alzheimer's disease prevalence.[1]

Tacrine (Cognex®), one of the most promoted dementia drugs in the United States, might reduce the "likelihood of nursing-home placement." But, as Dr. Pryse-Phillips reported, "the drug's adverse effects on the liver and high drop-out rate were recurrent problems. While tacrine is accepted in the United States and in some European countries, evaluation by the Canadian Health Protection Branch lead to its rejection on the grounds that the benefits did not translate into sufficient functional improvement to offset its potential risks (such as effects on the liver), an opinion strengthened by an assessment that concluded that it showed no clear evidence of efficacy or effectiveness."[4] In addition to Canada, several other countries have rejected tacrine, again because of its lack of clinical effectiveness and significant risk of potentially dangerous side effects.

The latest and most highly touted Alzheimer's drug, *donepezil* (Aricept®), has provided physicians yet another opportunity to convince themselves that they are "treating" a specific illness – in this case Alzheimer's disease. But the truth is that donepezil is essentially useless. As Dr. Pryse-Phillips reported, "Donepezil may improve certain neuro-psychological test scores, but its clinically meaningful benefits in treatment of Alzheimer's disease seem to be minimal."[5]

This revelation should hit home to prescribing physicians, especially in light of the potential for adverse reactions to this drug including depression, vomiting, dizziness, and insomnia.

What then explains the tens of thousands of prescriptions written each year for these drugs? The answer lies squarely in the over $5-billion spent by pharmaceutical companies promoting their wares. Pharmaceutical advertising targeted at physicians is so persuasive that the information presented is generally accepted as scientific fact. As an article in a recent *Consumer Reports* entitled *Pushing Drugs to Doctors* revealed, "A landmark 1982 study by Dr. Jerry Avorn of Harvard showed that doctors' opinions of two popular, heavily advertised drugs, came straight from the ads and sales pitches. The doctors believed they'd gotten their information from objective scientific sources, but those sources, in fact, had said all along that the drugs were not effective for their advertised uses."[6]

Our society focuses on treating medical problems with precious little attention paid to disease prevention. Indeed, it is the general purpose of this text to provide techniques designed to affect improvements in various neurodegenerative conditions, or at least slow the rate of an individual's decline. But it seems appropriate to first explore some of the emerging theories surrounding the causes of Alzheimer's disease.

Electromagnetic Fields

In these days of hand-held cellular phones, personal computers, and an abundance of other electronic devices, the general public seems to be at least marginally concerned about the possible health risks of electromagnetic radiation exposure as evidenced by articles appearing not only in alternative medical publications, but in mainstream journals as well.

In 1995, attention was drawn to the possible link between electromagnetic radiation and Alzheimer's disease following a landmark publication in the *American Journal of Epidemiology* by researchers at the *University of Southern California School of Medicine*.[7] Subsequently, these researchers confirmed a direct relationship between occupations exposing individuals to higher levels of electromagnetic radiation and the risk of developing Alzheimer's disease. Their report, published in the December 1996 issue of *Neurology*, revealed a substantial increased risk of developing Alzheimer's disease in individuals whose occupations exposed them to higher than average levels of electromagnetic radiation. The occupations determined to be "high risk" with respect to exposure included electrician, machinist, machine operator, seamstress, sewing factory worker, sheet metal worker, typist, keypunch operator, welder, machine shop worker, and several others. The risk of developing Alzheimer's disease in these individuals was calculated to be as much as *four times* higher

> *These researchers confirmed a direct relationship between occupations exposing individuals to higher levels of electromagnetic radiation and the risk of developing Alzheimer's disease.*

than the general population. Subjects evaluated were at least 65 years of age at the time of their first examination and their recorded occupations reflected what they had been doing up to 40 years prior to their evaluation and diagnosis of Alzheimer's disease.[8]

It is critical to recognize that the data used in this research reflected levels of electromagnetic exposure long before our population began using "cell-phones," personal computers, and the like.

How exposure to electronic devices may lead to Alzheimer's disease is unclear. Several authors have indicated that the electromagnetic radiation produced by electronic equipment enhances the formation of *beta amyloid*, a protein known to be prevalent in the brains of Alzheimer's patients.[9] Exactly how electromagnetic radiation increases beta amyloid is unclear, but it is clear that this protein enhances brain inflammation, now known to be the primary cause of brain degeneration in this disease.[10]

Perhaps because influences like electromagnetic radiation and toxic chemicals in the environment cannot be seen or perceived, there is reluctance by mainstream medicine to recognize potential health risks associated with these factors. Typically, when these topics are raised, a common response by defenders of the status quo seems to be "There is no peer reviewed literature supporting these outlandish claims." But in reality, that is simply not the case. The journal in which this research was published is the "*Official Journal of the American Academy of Neurology*," perhaps the most well respected peer reviewed journal dealing with neurologic disease in the world. Somehow it seems that articles linking environmental factors with disease, much like research dealing with the impact of nutrition on health, are generally overlooked in favor of concentrating on pharmaceutical approaches to treating the illnesses they cause.

Aluminum

Another generally unnoticed but certainly important risk factor for the development of Alzheimer's disease is exposure to aluminum. This relationship has not escaped the eyes of the manufacturers of various consumer products as we now see a proliferation of advertisements for everything from aluminum-free antiperspirants and shampoos, to ads claiming a specific antacid is better than the next as it contains "no aluminum." But is the threat of aluminum anything more than what we read in health-food store shopping bag stuffers?

In actuality, the science relating Alzheimer's and aluminum appears in our most highly respected medical journals. Reporting in the journal *Neurology* in 1996, researchers from the *University of Toronto* found an astounding 250% increased risk of Alzheimer's disease in individuals drinking municipal water high in aluminum for a 10 or more year period of time. Alzheimer's risk increased by 70% in those exposed to municipal drinking water containing only minimally increased amounts of aluminum – water consumed by an alarming 19% of the Ontario population. Based upon their findings and the many scientific reports of elevated levels of aluminum in the brains of Alzheimer's patients, the authors concluded, " The findings from epidemiological studies, coupled with the large body of experimental evidence of aluminum neurotoxicity and elevated concentration in Alzheimer's disease affected brain, argue that priority should be given to consideration of lowering, and maintaining, acceptable limits of residual aluminum in drinking water ... particularly for older age groups at risk for Alzheimer's disease."[11]

Alzheimer's risk increased by 70% in those exposed to municipal drinking water containing only minimally increased amounts of aluminum.

One could certainly argue the rationale for reducing aluminum exposure "particularly for older age groups at risk for Alzheimer's disease" since aluminum accumulates over many years regardless of age, and we will all be members of the "older age group" eventually. But nevertheless, studies like these are a wake-up call alerting us that diseases like Alzheimer's are not random events, but are, at least to some degree, diseases brought about by factors over which we have control.

The likelihood of Alzheimer's disease being related to aluminum is further strengthened by a report in the journal *The Lancet* which described actual slowing of progression of dementia in Alzheimer's disease following administration of *desferoximine*, a chemical known to enhance aluminum excretion.[12]

How aluminum increases Alzheimer's risk is now fairly well understood. Like other metals, aluminum directly enhances the formation of dangerous free radicals, leading to progressive damage of the delicate cell membranes surrounding neurons.[13] Eventually, this cumulative damage hampers neuronal function which manifests as failure in such areas as memory and reasoning – characteristics commonly associated with Alzheimer's disease.

The damaging effects of free radicals produced by the presence of aluminum can be significantly reduced by the administration of *melatonin*, a powerful brain antioxidant.[14] Melatonin is produced by the pineal gland, a small almond shaped structure situated in the back of the brain. The production of this important hormone rapidly declines with age. In addition, melatonin production is extremely light sensitive, being produced almost exclusively during darkness.

 In an intriguing report from South Africa, researchers tried to explain why Alzheimer's disease is exceedingly rare in rural Africa, while prevalent in more developed areas. They reasoned that, "Since melatonin is produced by the pineal gland only in the dark, the excess of electric light in developed countries may help explain why Alzheimer's disease is more prevalent in these countries than in rural Africa."[15]

In an article appearing in the *Townsend Letter for Doctors* in 1993, Dr. Michael A. Weiner, executive director of the *Alzheimer's Research Institute* summarized our present understanding of the dangers of aluminum exposure stating, "aluminum has been known as a neurotoxic substance for nearly a century. The scientific literature on its toxic effects has now grown to a critical mass. It is not necessary to conclude that aluminum causes Alzheimer's disease to recommend that it be reduced or eliminated as a potential risk. It is the only element noted to accumulate in the tangle-bearing neurons characteristic of the disease and is also found in elevated amounts in four regions of the brain of Alzheimer's patients."[16]

Aluminum has been known as a neurotoxic substance for nearly a century.

Aside from municipal drinking water, other potential sources for aluminum exposure are many and include nondairy creamers, self-rising flours, cake mixes, and various processed foods, especially individually wrapped cheese slices. We are able to excrete about 20 milligrams of ingested aluminum each day,[17] but this amount can be greatly exceeded by even a single antacid tablet which may provide as much as 200 milligrams of aluminum. Other medications high in aluminum include many buffered analgesic products. A list of various aluminum containing medications is found at the end of this chapter.

Homocysteine

In this context, efforts aimed at preventing dementia would certainly seem to take on more importance. In an interesting report appearing in the *Lancet,* May 8, 1999, from the *Department of Neurology and Clinical Chemistry at the University of Heidelberg,* researchers revealed that the second most frequent cause of dementia in the elderly population after Alzheimer's disease was so called "vascular dementia," or brain dysfunction as a consequence of disease of the small blood vessels (see chapter 6). What was more striking, was the finding of elevation of a particular chemical in the blood of these individuals called *homocysteine.*[18] Blood homocysteine levels are directly related to intake of the B-complex group of vitamins, specifically, vitamins B6, and B12, as well as folic acid. The conclusion of the report provided very strong support for the effectiveness of dietary supplementation with the B-complex group of vitamins in terms of reducing risk of dementia. As the author stated "We speculate, therefore,

Researchers noted a 200% increased risk of Alzheimer's disease in individuals with elevation of blood homocysteine levels.

that progression of vascular dementia in patients with identified hyperhomocysteinemia (elevated homocysteine) could be prevented by vitamin supplementation."[19]

But apart from vascular dementia, elevation of homocysteine has even more important implications. New research has found that elevation of this blood chemical is directly related to the risk of Alzheimer's disease – the most common dementing illness. In a 1998 article published in *Archives of Neurology*, researchers noted a 200% increased risk of Alzheimer's disease in individuals with elevation of blood homocysteine levels.[20] And again, elevated homocysteine can almost always be normalized with simple vitamin therapy!

More distressing is the fact that levels of brain damaging homocysteine can be increased by some commonly used medications including L-dopa[21] (Sinemet®), the mainstay treatment for Parkinson's disease, as well as antibiotics containing trimethoprim[22] (Bactrim® and Septra®).

Inflammation

While the idea that the process of inflammation accounts for the tissue destruction in diseases like arthritis is widely recognized, accepting the role for inflammation in Alzheimer's is somehow more difficult. Nevertheless, the current understanding of Alzheimer's disease holds that:

Symptoms of Alzheimer's disease result from failure of neurons damaged or destroyed by free radicals generated by inflammation.[23]

This thesis is supported by many studies demonstrating higher levels of inflammation specific chemicals known as *cytokines* in brains of Alzheimer's patients, as well as the finding of reduced risk of the disease in individuals having a history of treatment with the common class of arthritis medicines known as nonsteroidal anti-inflammatory drugs (NSAIDs) or aspirin.[24] In a 1997 publication in the journal *Neurology*, researchers from the *Johns Hopkins School of Medicine* reported a relative risk of Alzheimer's disease of only 40% of normal in individuals reporting 2 or more years of using NSAIDs. Risk was 74% of normal in aspirin users, while there was an actual *increase* in risk of Alzheimer's (35% above normal) in the group taking acetaminophen (the active ingredient in Tylenol®) for two years or more.[25] Why acetaminophen might actually increase the risk of

Alzheimer's disease may relate to its effect on an important antioxidant, *glutathione*. Glutathione serves as one of the primary brain antioxidants so its deficiency could potentially allow increased free radical damage. Acetaminophen has been shown to reduce glutathione production, thus paving the way for enhanced brain destruction by free radicals.[26]

The role of inflammation in Alzheimer's goes far beyond simple consideration of whether someone has taken a specific arthritis drug in the past or not. Inflammation may actually represent the

Acetaminophen has been shown to reduce glutathione production, thus paving the way for enhanced brain destruction by free radicals.

mechanism linking specific dietary patterns to either the development of the disease or enhancing its progression. In a compelling 1998 report appearing in the journal *Medical Hypothesis* entitled *"Could diet be used to reduce the risk of Alzheimer's disease?,"* Dr. P.E. Newman describes how a specific breakdown product of dietary fat, *arachidonic acid,* profoundly enhances inflammation.[27] Indeed, it is the inhibition of the formation of arachidonic acid that explains the function of various anti-inflammatory drugs. Dr. Newman then reveals how other dietary fats, namely the essential fatty acids from the omega-3 and omega-6 groups, have just the opposite effect – they actually reduce the inflammatory process.

Inflammation causing arachidonic acid is found in abundance in meats, meat products, and eggs. It is efficiently absorbed from the gut and is incorporated into the membranes of cells more readily than any other fatty acid. As Dr. Newman stated, " It has been estimated that persons eating a

Inflammation causing arachidonic acid is found in abundance in meats, meat products, and eggs.

typical Western diet take in between 200 and 100 mg per day of arachidonic acid in their food. As the normal requirement of arachidonic acid is only about 1 mg per day... it is easy to understand why over the years persons in the industrialized countries build up excessive pools of arachidonic acid and why older persons in such societies tend to develop ...rheumatoid arthritis, atherosclerosis, certain neoplasms (cancers), psoriasis, and why not, Alzheimer's disease."[28]

This offers a strong and sound argument against meat and egg consumption, and supports the use of essential fatty acid supplements (see below) combined with diets rich in fish, vegetables and grains - natural sources of the inflammation reducing omega-3 and omega-6 oils.

Powerful Therapy

Effective therapy for Alzheimer's disease must accomplish three tasks – reduce inflammation, limit the damaging effects of free radicals, and enhance neuronal function.

Reducing Inflammation

Essential Fatty Acids

Manipulation of dietary fats is a proven therapy to reduce inflammation. Dietary changes designed to reduce arachidonic acid (less meat and eggs), while increasing omega-3 and omega-6 levels have been demonstrated to be effective in a variety of inflammatory conditions including arthritis, psoriasis and multiple sclerosis (see chapter 2). This is why essential fatty acid supplementation is an integral part of the **BrainRecovery.com** protocol for Alzheimer's disease. The best source for omega-3 fats are fish oils, the potency of which is determined by its DHA content. Flaxseed oil is another source for omega-3's, but provides considerably less DHA compared to supplements derived from fish oil.

The best sources for omega-6 oils are borage seed oil and evening primrose oil. Potency of the omega-6 group is determined by the content of GLA. Zinc, magnesium, and vitamins B3 and B6 enhance the anti-inflammatory effects of both of these essential fatty acids. An accurate level of both the inflammation enhancing fatty acids and those which reduce this activity can be easily assessed using a simple blood test, the *Essential Fatty Acid Panel,* from Great Smokies Diagnostic Laboratory in Asheville, North Carolina (see below).

Limiting Free Radical Activity

Vitamin E

The utilization of antioxidants to limit the activity of free radicals as therapy for Alzheimer's disease has been extensively evaluated over the past decade. Perhaps the most widely studied is vitamin E – a good candidate not only because of its powerful antioxidant activity, but also because of its high fat solubility. This feature is crucial since not only is the brain more than 60% fat, but it is the fat component that is at highest risk for free radical damage.

The group taking vitamin E did best in all areas including longevity and cognitive function – better than the prescription medication.

Based upon these characteristics, vitamin E would seem the ideal candidate for Alzheimer's disease therapy and as such was the subject of a landmark study published in the *New England Journal of Medicine* in 1997. In this study, patients were given Vitamin E, selegiline (another so-called "Alzheimer's drug"), both, or placebo for two years.

At the end of the study data was compiled assessing such parameters as being institutionalized, loss of ability to perform activities of self-care, "severe" dementia, and death. The compelling results clearly demonstrated that the group taking vitamin E did best in all areas including longevity and cognitive function – *better than the prescription medication.*[29]

The other important role for vitamin E is that it serves to protect dietary essential fatty acids from being rendered less effective by oxidation. Vitamin E must always be included in any nutritional program utilizing essential fatty acid supplementation as described above.

Gingko biloba

The therapeutic use of Gingko biloba goes back centuries and is described in traditional Chinese pharmacopoeia. In France, extracts of Gingko biloba are administered orally and intravenously and are among the most commonly prescribed pharmaceutical drugs as they are in Germany where Ginkgo is licensed for the treatment of a variety of brain disorders including headache, tinnitus, vertigo and memory disorders.

Perhaps the most convincing validation of the effectiveness of Ginkgo biloba comes from a 1997 publication entitled "*A Placebo-Controlled, Double-blind, Randomized Trial of an Extract of Ginkgo Biloba for Dementia,*" published in none other than the *Journal of the American Medical Association*. In this study, the progress of over 200 Alzheimer's patients was evaluated over a 1-year period. Half the group received Ginkgo biloba, while the other half received a placebo. The results were dramatic. At the completion of the study, the placebo group showed a progressive decline in mental function on a standardized psychological test while the group receiving Ginkgo, on average, actually *improved*. Similar results were also noted in independent evaluations of social skills. The authors concluded that Ginkgo biloba was, "safe and appears capable of stabilizing and, in a substantial number of cases, improving the cognitive performance and the social functioning of demented patients for 6 months to 1 year."[30]

The effectiveness of Gingko biloba may be explained by several mechanisms including increasing blood flow, improving cerebral metabolism, and perhaps most importantly, its antioxidant potential, reducing the damaging activity of free radicals.[31]

Alpha Lipoic Acid

In the next decade, lipoic acid will clearly rank as one of the most important discoveries in the treatment of neurodegenerative diseases. New research is being published almost every day describing the vast potential of this nutrient, and with good reason. Lipoic acid is a powerful anti-oxidant that is rapidly absorbed from the gut and readily enters the brain to protect neurons from free radical damage. Further antioxidant protection is derived from its ability to recycle vitamins C and E, and regenerate *glutathione*, one of the brain's most important antioxidants.

The brains of Alzheimer's patients have been shown to contain significantly elevated levels of iron, a "catalyst" which enhances free radical production.[32] Lipoic acid acts as a powerful metal chelator. It binds several potentially toxic metals in the body including cadmium and free iron, and facilitates their excretion. This is another important reason why lipoic acid is part of the **BrainRecovery.com** protocol for Alzheimer's disease.

N-Acetyl-Cysteine (NAC)

As mentioned above, glutathione is one of the most important brain antioxidants. Deficiency of glutathione activity has been described in various neurodegenerative conditions. To be effective, glutathione must be administered intravenously as described in chapter one. Fortunately, glutathione production can be enhanced by the oral administration of NAC.

In addition to increasing glutathione, NAC has an important antioxidant role in and of itself. One of the most notorious free radicals implicated in Alzheimer's disease is *nitric oxide*. Nitric oxide is formed by the activation of an enzyme, *nitric oxide synthase*. NAC has the unique ability to reduce the activity of nitric oxide synthase and thus reduce the generation of nitric oxide.[33] The overall effect is a marked lowering of free radical activity, thus creating a less hostile environment for delicate brain tissue.

Vitamin D

Typically regarded as having utility only in preserving bone density, vitamin D has recently been demonstrated to have profound antioxidant activity. Like vitamin E, it is highly fat soluble, making it an ideal candidate as a brain protecting

Moderate to severe deficiencies of vitamin D were found in 80% of Alzheimer's patients studied.

free radical scavenger. In fact, vitamin D has been shown to have even more potency as an antioxidant when compared to vitamin E. Remarkably, in a Japanese study published in 1998, it was found that moderate to severe deficiencies of vitamin D were found in 80% of Alzheimer's patients studied. Unfortunately, the authors failed to recognize the potency of vitamin D as an antioxidant and focused their comments exclusively on its role in bone health.[34]

Enhancing Neuronal Function

Coenzyme Q10 (CoQ10)

Coenzyme Q10 is a critical transporter of electrons in the process of energy production in every living cell. As such, deficiencies of CoQ10 function have profound effects on cellular activity and viability. CoQ10 supplementation has been demonstrated to enhance energy

CoQ10 supplementation has been demonstrated to enhance energy production in brain neurons and thus improve function.

production in brain neurons and thus improve function.[35] In addition, new research demonstrates a direct correlation between CoQ10 levels and longevity in a variety of animal species.[36] This likely stems not only from CoQ10's role in enhancing energy production, but its significant antioxidant activity as well. Isn't it then critically important to recognize that two of the most widely prescribed cholesterol lowering drugs, pravastatin (Pravachol®) and lovastatin (Mevacor®), can significantly lower serum coenzyme Q10 levels?[37]

Nicotinamide Adenine Dinucleotide (NADH)

Like CoQ10, NADH is both an essential ingredient for the chemical reactions powering all living cells and a powerful antioxidant. Because defects of cellular energy production and free radical damage are two of the fundamental mechanisms underlying Alzheimer's disease, NADH would seem to be a perfect candidate for clinical study. In a 1996 article appearing in *Annals of Clinical and Laboratory Science*, Dr. Jörg Birkmayer reported a significant improvement in cognitive performance as measured on a standardized mental performance test in a group of Alzheimer's patients given NADH. Those not receiving the supplement continued to deteriorate. Dr. Birkmayer noted that in addition to increasing cellular energy production, NADH also enhanced the production of two important brain chemicals, *dopamine* and *noradrenaline* – both noted to be deficient in Alzheimer's patients. As he stated, " The concept of using NADH as an anti-dementia agent follows a strategy which differs from the approaches mentioned previously. The NADH seems to act in two ways. One is the stimulation of the endogenous biosynthesis of dopamine and noradrenaline. The other is an increase in energy production of cells in the brain and in the periphery."[38]

Acetyl-L-carnitine

Acetyl-L-carnitine functions primarily as a shuttle, transporting critical fuel sources into the *mitochondria*, the energy producing machinery of the neuron. Its second task is to facilitate the removal of the toxic byproducts of brain metabolism. Because of these functions, acetyl-L-carnitine has a pivotal role in facilitating the fundamental processes necessary for brain cell survival.

In addition, acetyl-L-carnitine is readily converted into an important *neurotransmitter* (brain chemical messenger) known as *acetylcholine,* which is known to be profoundly deficient in the brains of Alzheimer's patients.

It is for these reasons that acetyl-L-carnitine has been so extensively evaluated in dementia studies. In a report entitled *"A 1-year multicenter placebo-controlled study of acetyl-L-carnitine in patients with Alzheimer's disease"* which appeared in the journal *Neurology*, researchers at the University of California, San Diego found a striking reduction in the rate of mental decline in younger Alzheimer's patients taking acetyl-L-carnitine over the 1 year evaluation.[39]

> *Researchers found a striking reduction in the rate of mental decline in younger Alzheimer's patients taking acetyl-L-carnitine over the 1 year evaluation.*

Phosphatidylserine

Over the past 2 decades extensive medical literature has appeared describing the important role of *lecithin* in preserving normal brain function. More recent research has revealed that the beneficial action of lecithin is, for the most part, due to one of its components, phosphatidylserine.

Phosphatidylserine is one of the key constituents of *neuronal membranes* - the site where brain cells both receive and transmit chemical messages. Abnormalities of the neuronal membrane have been linked to age-related functional changes in brain performance. Another important membrane in nerve cells requiring adequate phosphatidylserine is that which surrounds the energy producing structures, the mitochondria. Adequate phosphatidylserine is a basic requirement to maintain vital energy production of the mitochondria, ensuring optimal function of the brain.

These important functions of phosphatidylserine have prompted vigorous research into its therapeutic potential in dementia. In a 1991 article entitled *"Effects of phosphatidylserine in age-associated memory impairment,"* appearing in the journal *Neurology*, researchers from *Stanford University* treated 149 memory impaired patients with phosphatidylserine for 12 weeks and observed a marked improvement on performance tests related to memory and learning compared to a similar group receiving a placebo. The authors stated, "These results suggest that the compound may be a promising candidate for treating memory loss in later life."[40]

Vitamin B-12

Patients suffering from Alzheimer's disease generally have significantly lower blood levels of vitamin B-12.

Standard medical texts have long reported that vitamin B-12 is a critical factor for preservation of normal brain function. Its deficiency is associated with confusion, depression, mental slowness, memory difficulties, and abnormalities of nerve function. Several studies have demonstrated that patients suffering from Alzheimer's disease generally have significantly lower blood levels of vitamin B-12 compared to age matched, non-afflicted individuals.[41] Perhaps its most important function is its role in the maintenance of myelin, the protective, insulating coat surrounding each neuron. New research reveals that B12 helps prevent the accumulation of the brain damaging amino acid *homocysteine*, which, when elevated, markedly increases the risk for Alzheimer's disease as described above.

Folic Acid

Folic acid levels are often markedly depressed in patients suffering from dementia or confusional states. Deficiency of folic acid is associated with apathy, disorientation, memory deficits, and difficulties with concentration. Several studies have correlated low folic acid levels with dementia.[42] Again, the mechanism may involve elevation of homocysteine since like vitamin B12, folic acid helps lower this blood vessel damaging amino acid.

BrainRecovery.com – Alzheimer's Disease Summary

The science relating electromagnetic radiation exposure to Alzheimer's disease is sound. Reducing the risk of Alzheimer's disease involves a recognition and avoidance of potential sources of electromagnetic radiation like hand-held cellular telephones, electric blankets, hand-held hair dryers, clock-radios on the night stand near the head, and desktop computers, to name but a few.

The relationship between Alzheimer's disease and aluminum is supported by several observations including worldwide epidemiological reports, the presence of extremely high brain aluminum levels in Alzheimer's patients, and studies revealing that aluminum increases damaging free radicals. Many municipal water utilities add aluminum sulfate to public water sources to help remove fine particulate matter. This is a strong argument in favor of drinking bottled water. Avoid medications containing aluminum (see below). Read ingredient labels of food products to help avoid aluminum consumption. Food cooked in aluminum cookware can absorb substantial amounts of aluminum. Choose glass or stainless steel. And remember that melatonin can limit aluminum's damaging effects.

Avoid medications containing acetaminophen as it reduces the availability of the important antioxidant glutathione. Research shows increased risk of Alzheimer's in those taking acetaminophen with decreased risk in individuals choosing nonsteroidal anti-inflammatory drugs or aspirin. So choose Advil® or aspirin over Tylenol® as an analgesic.

Meat and eggs are rich inflammation producing fatty acids. And it is this inflammation that leads to the enhanced production of brain damaging free radicals. The best diet is vegetarian with added fish. Supplementation with oils rich in appropriate essential fatty acids can remarkably reduce inflammation - reducing free radical production.

Appropriate antioxidants and cellular energizers, substantiated by research published in the most well respected scientific and medical journals, have important roles in any treatment plan for this disease.

BrainRecovery.com
Alzheimer's Protocol

Vitamin B12 _____ 1cc (1000mcg) injected IM daily
for 5 days, then twice weekly (see above)

Essential fatty acids: <u>daily dose</u>
   Linolenic acid
      EPA / DHA fish oil providing _____ DHA 500 mg
     (see note below)
    and

   Linoleic acid
      Evening Primrose oil, or
      Borage oil, or
      Black Currant oil providing _____ GLA 300 mg

Vitamins and Antioxidants

Vitamin B3	100 mg
Vitamin B6	100 mg
Vitamin C	800 mg
Vitamin E	400 IU
Alpha lipoic acid	80 mg
N-Acetyl Cysteine	400 mg
Ginkgo Biloba	60 mg
Vitamin D	400 IU
Melatonin	3 mg at bedtime

Cellular Energizers

Coenzyme Q10 _____ 60 mg
NADH _____ 5 mg (twice daily)
Phosphatidylserine _____ 100 mg
Acetyl-L-carnitine _____ 400 mg

Minerals

Magnesium _____ 400 mg
Zinc _____ 20 mg

Or, if using the Brain Sustain™ supplement:

Vitamin B12 by injection essential fatty acids, NADH
and melatonin as above, and:

Brain Sustain™ _____ 2 scoops daily

Note:

The highest quality DHA containing fish oil supplements are manufactured by **Nordic Naturals, Inc.,** and are available by calling
i **Nutritionals** at: 1-800-530-1982 or by visiting the website
www.BrainRecovery.com

ANTACIDS WITH ALUMINUM

Maalox tablets
Mintox Tablets
RuLox #1 tablets
RuLox #2 Tablets
Extra Strength Maalox Tablets
Acid-X
Duracid Tablets
Titralac Extra Strength Tablets
Marblen Tablets
Alkets Tablets
Mi-Acid Gelcaps
Mylanta Gelcaps
Myalgen Gelcaps
Calglycine Antacid
Titralac Tablets
Alenic Alka Tablets

Foamicon Tablets
Genaton Tablets
Gaviscon Tablets
Double Strength Gaviscon-2 Tablets
Extra Strength Alenic Alka Tablets
Extra Strength Genaton Tablets
Almacone Tablets
Mylanta Tablets
RuLoxPlus Tablets
Magalox Plus
Gelusil Tablets
Maalox Plus Tablets
Mintox Plus Tablets
Extra Strength Maalox Plus Tablets
Mylanta Double Strength Tablets
Tempo Tablets

ANALGESICS WITH ALUMINUM

Buffets II Tablets
Vanquish Caplets
Cope Tablets

ANALGESICS WITHOUT ALUMINUM

Bayer Select Maximum Strength Headache Caplets
Anacin Caplets and Tablets
Anacin Maximum Strength Tablets

From: Drug Facts and Comparisons, ® 1999 Edition
Published by Facts and Comparisons ®
111 West Port Plaza, Suite 300
St. Louis, MO 63146-3098

BrainSustain is a nutritional supplement designed to maintain healthy brain function. It is not intended to treat or cure any specific disease.

Resources

1. The 36-Hour Day: A Family Guide to Caring for Persons with Alzheimer Disease, Related Dementing Illnesses, and Memory Loss in Later Life, Third Edition, by Nancy L. MacE, Peter V. Rabins, Paul R. McHugh.1999, Johns Hopkins Univ Pr; ISBN: 0801861497

References

[1] Cumings J.L., Current Perspectives in Alzheimer's disease. Neurology 51 (suppl. 1): S1,1998

[2] Martin, J.B., Molecular Basis of the Neurodegenerative Disorders. N Eng J Med 340(25): 1970-80,1999

[3] Pryse-Phillips, W., Do We Have Drugs for Dementia? Arch Neurol 56:735-737, 1999

[4] Ibid.

[5] Ibid.

[6] Avorn, J., In: *Pushing Drugs to Doctors.* Consumer Reports,Feb.: p 88,1992

[7] Sobel, E., Davanipour, Z., Sulkave, R., et al., Occupations with exposure to electromagnetic fields: a possible risk factor for Alzheimer's disease. Am J Epidemiol 142:515-524, 1995

[8] Sobel, E., Dunn, M., Davanipour, Z., et al., Elevated risk of Alzheimer's disease among workers with likely electromagnetic field exposure. Neurology 47:1477-81, 1996

[9] 1594

[10] Floyd, R.A., Neuroinflammatory Processes are Important in Neurodegenerative Diseases: An Hypothesis to Explain the Increased Formation of Reactive Oxygen and Nitrogen Species as Major Factors Involved in Neurodegenerative Disease Development. Free Radical Biology and Medicine 26 (9/10): 1346-55, 1999

[11] McLachlan, D.R.C., Bergeron, C., Smith, J.E., et al., Risk for Neuropathologically confirmed Alzheimer's disease and residual aluminum in municipal drinking water employing weighted residential histories. Neurology 46: 401-405, 1996

[12] Crapper McLachlan, D.R., Dalton, A.J., Kruck, T.P. et al., Intramuscular desferrioxamine in patients with Alzheimer's disease. Lancet 337(8753): 1304-1308, 1991

[13] Janetzky, B., Reichmann, H., Youdim, M.B.H., Iron and Oxidative Damage in Neurodegenerative Diseases, in *Mitochondria and Free Radicals in Neurodegenerative Diseases.* Beal, M.F.(ed.),New York, Wiley-Liss Pub. 1997

[14] Daniels, W.M., van Rensberg, S.J., van Zyl, J.M., et al., Melatonin prevents beta-amyloid induced lipid peroxidation. J Pineal Res 24(2):78-82, 1998

[15] van Rensberg, S.J., Daniels, W.M., Potocnik, F.C., et al., A new model for the pathophysiology of Alzheimer's disease. Aluminum toxicity is exacerbated by hydrogen peroxide and attenuated by an amyloid protein fragment and melatonin. S Afr J Med 87(9):1111-1115, 1997

[16] Weiner, M.A., Evidence points to aluminum's link with Alzheimer's disease. Townsend Letter for Doctors 124:1103, 1993

[17] Birchall, J.D., Chappel, J.S., Aluminum, Chemical Physiology and Alzheimer's Disease. Lancet 2(8618):1008-10, 1988

[18] Faâender, K., Mielke, O., Bertsch, T., et al., Homocysteine in cerebral macroangiography and microangiopathy.Lancet 3531586-87, 1999

[19] Ibid.

[20] Clarke, R., Smith, A.D., Jobst, K.A., et al, Folate, vitamin B12, and serum total homocysteine levels in confirmed Alzheimer's disease. Arch Neurol 55:1449-55, 1998

[21] Müller, T., Werne, B., Fowler, W., et al., Nigral endothelial dysfunction and Parkinson's disease. Lancet 354, 126-127, 1999

[22] Smulders, Y.M., de Man, A.M.E., Stehouwer, C.D.A., Trimethoprim and fasting homocysteine. Lancet 352:1827-28, 1998

[23] Floyd, R.A., Neuroinflammatory Processes are Important in Neurodegenerative Diseases: An Hypothesis to Explain the Increased Formation of Reactive Oxygen and Nitrogen Species as Major Factors Involved in Neurodegenerative Disease Development. Free Radical Biology and Medicine 26 (9/10): 1346-55, 1999

[24] Ibid.

[25] Stewart, W.F., Kawas, C., Corrada, M., Risk of Alzheimer's disease and duration of NSAID use. Neurology 48: 626-632, 1997

[26] Vendemiale, G., Grattagliano, I., Altomare, E., et al., Effect of acetaminophen on hepatic glutathione compartmentation and mitochondrial energy metabolism in the rat. Biochem Pharmacol 25:52 (8): 1147-54, 1996

[27] Newman, P.E., Could diet be used to reduce the risk of developing Alzheimer's disease? Med Hypothesis 50:335-37, 1998

[28] Ibid.

[29] Sano, M., Ernesto, C., Thomas, R.G., et al., A controlled trial of selegeline, alpha-tocopherol, or both as treatment for Alzheimer's disease. N Engl J Med 336:1216-22, 1997

[30] Le Bars, P., Katz, M.M., Berman, N., et al., A Placebo-Controlled, Double-blind Randomized Trial of an Extract of Ginkgo Biloba for Dementia. JAMA 278(16):1327-32,1997

[31] Ibid.

[32] Janetzky, B., Reichmann, H., Youdim, M.B.H., Iron and Oxidative Damage in Neurodegenerative Diseases, in *Mitochondria and Free Radicals in Neurodegenerative Diseases.* Beal, M.F.(ed.),New York, Wiley-Liss Pub. 1997

[33] Pahan, J., Sheikh, F.G., Namboodiri, A.M.S., N-acetyl cysteine inhibits induction of NO production by endotoxin or cytokine stimulated rat peritoneal macrophages, C6 glial cells and astrocytes. Free Radical Biology and Medicine 24(1): 39-48, 1997

[34] Stao, Y., Asoh, T., Oizumi, K., High prevalence of vitamin D deficiency and reduced bone mass in elderly women with Alzheimer's disease. Bone 23(6):555-557, 1998

[35] Shults, C.W., Beal, M.F., Fontaine, K. et al., Absorption, tolerability and effects on mitochondrial activity of oral coenzyme Q10 in parkinsonian patients. Neurology 50: 793-795,1998

[36] Lass, A., Sohal, R.S., Comparisons of Coenzyme Q bound to mitochondrial membrane proteins among different mammalian species. Free Radical Biology and Medicine 27(1/2):220-26,1999

[37] Mortensen, S.A., Leth, A., Agner, E., Dose-related decrease of serum coenzyme Q10 during treatment with HMG-CoA reductase inhibitors. Mol Aspects of Med 18(Suppl.) S137-44, 1997

[38] Birkmayer, J.G.D., Coenzyme Nicotinamide Adenine Dinucleotide – New Therapeutic Approach for Improving Dementia of the Alzheimer Type. Ann Clin and Lab Science 26(1):1-9, 1996

[39] Thal, L.J., Carta, A., Clarke, W.R., et al., A 1-year multicenter placebo-controlled study of acetyl-L-carnitine in patients with Alzheimer's disease. Neurology 47:705-711, 1996

[40] Crook, T.H., Tinklenberg, J., Yesavage, J., Effects of phosphatidylserine in age-associated memory impairment. Neurology 41:644-49, 1991

[41] Clarke, R., Smith, A.D., Jobst, K.A., et al, Folate, vitamin B12, and serum total homocysteine levels in confirmed Alzheimer's disease. Arch Neurol 55:1449-55, 1998

[42] Ibid.

CHAPTER SIX

Vascular Dementia

Vascular dementia is a common cause of dementia in the elderly, second only to Alzheimer's disease in frequency. Unlike Alzheimer's disease, the process leading to brain tissue destruction in vascular dementia is well understood. In this disease, the critical damaging factor centers on compromised blood supply. Damage to the small blood vessels supplying the brain leads to a progressive decline in function with patients frequently becoming severely demented.

When confronted with dementia, several factors in the patient's history and physical examination help differentiate vascular dementia from Alzheimer's disease. This distinction is important since the treatment approaches to these two diseases differ significantly. Factors favoring the diagnosis of vascular dementia are noted in table 6.1.

The last factor, homocysteine, is an amino acid now known to be directly related to increased risk for various vascular conditions including myocardial infarction and stroke. In a recent report in the journal *The Lancet*, German researchers revealed a striking relationship between elevation of blood homocysteine and risk of vascular dementia[1]. This has profound implications both from a disease prevention perspective as well as for treatment strategies designed to slow the progression of the disease since elevation of homocysteine is often a reflection of vitamin deficiency.

Table 6.1. Characteristics of vascular dementia
abrupt onset
stepwise progression
nocturnal confusion
preservation of personality
depression
evidence of other vascular disease difficulty controlling emotions
hypertension
history of stroke
elevated homocysteine

Specifically, deficiencies of vitamins B6, B12 and folic acid are known to greatly increase the risk of homocysteine elevation and therefore increase the risk of vascular dementia. That is to say that simple attention to vitamin supplementation could have profound implications in terms of reducing the risk of a devastating disease. Further, identifying "at-risk" individuals requires nothing more than a simple blood test to evaluate homocysteine status (see below). Once identified, elevated homocysteine can almost always be brought down to normal levels with a simple nonprescription vitamin program. This lack of requirement of a pharmaceutical intervention to correct elevated homocysteine may explain why the general public has remained in the dark about this easily modifiable risk factor.

Vinpocetine

Vinpocetine is an extract of the periwinkle plant, *Vinca minor*. Its discovery has essentially revolutionized the treatment of vascular dementia.

In humans, vinpocetine has been demonstrated to increase brain blood flow, reduce

Vinpocetine has been demonstrated to increase brain blood flow, reduce blood viscosity, increase brain metabolism, and act as a potent antioxidant.

blood viscosity, increase brain metabolism, and act as a potent antioxidant.[2,3] These actions have prompted extensive research to evaluate the efficacy of vinpocetine in the treatment of vascular dementia.

In a 1987 study published in the Journal of the *American Geriatric Society*, Italian researches confirmed the effectiveness of vinpocetine in treating vascular dementia. Their report stated, "The overall clinical judgment of the effectiveness of treatment, made by the investigator at the end of the study, assessed 56% of the patients in the vinpocetine group as having made good to excellent improvement since entering the study." And further, " Patients on vinpocetine scored consistently better than placebo patients in all evaluations of the effectiveness of treatment"[4] Their results have consistently been confirmed by other researchers.[5]

BrainRecovery.com
Vascular Dementia Protocol

The BrainRecovery.com protocol for vascular dementia is similar to that described for Alzheimer's disease in that both entities require techniques designed to both protect the brain from free radical damage as well as enhance energy production (metabolism) in the surviving brain neurons. It is the addition of vinpocetine and special attention to identifying and treating elevated homocysteine that are unique features of the vascular dementia protocol.

Vitamins and Antioxidants

	daily dose
Vitamin B3	100 mg
Vitamin B6	100 mg
Vitamin C	800 mg
Vitamin E	400 IU
Alpha lipoic acid	80 mg
N-Acetyl Cysteine	400 mg
Ginkgo Biloba	60 mg
Vitamin D	400 IU
Folic acid	800mcg
Vitamin B12	200mcg

Cellular Energizers

Coenzyme Q10	60 mg
NADH	5 mg (twice daily)
Phosphatidylserine	100 mg
Acetyl-L-carnitine	400 mg

Or, if using the Brain Sustain™ supplement:

Vinpocetine 5mg twice daily, and :

Brain Sustain™ _____ 2 scoops daily

Vitamin B12 _____ 1000mcg
(if homocysteine elevated)

Homocysteine can be evaluated by having your doctor or lab send a blood sample to:

Great Smokies Diagnostic Laboratory
63 Zillicoa Street
Asheville, N.C. 28801-9801
Tel. (800) 522 – 4762

BrainSustain is a nutritional supplement designed to maintain healthy brain function. It is not intended to treat or cure any specific disease.

References

[1] Fabender, K., Mielke, O., Bertsh, T., et al., Homocysteine in cerebral macroangiography and microangiopathy. Lancet 353:1586-87,1999

[2] Tamaki, N., Kusunoki, T., Matsumoto, S., The effect of Vinpocetine on cerebral blood flow in patients with cerebrovascular disease. Ther Hung , 33: 13-21. 1985

[3] Olah, V.A. Balla, G., Balla, J., et al., An in vitro study of the hydroxyl scavenger effect of caviton. Acta Paediatr Hung, 30: 309-316, 1990

[4] Balestreri, R., Fontana, L., and Astengo, F., A double-blind placebo controlled evaluation of the safety and efficacy of vinpocetine in the treatment of patients with chronic vascular senile cerebral dysfunction. J Am Geriatr Soc 35: 425-430, 1987

[5] Hindmarch, I., Fuchs, H., Erzigkeit, H., Efficacy and tolerance of vinpocetine in ambulant patients suffering from mild to moderate organic psychosyndromes. Int Clin Psychopharmacol 6: 31-43, 1991

CHAPTER SEVEN

Stroke Recovery

It has been estimated that in the United States there are at present approximately 1.7 million stroke survivors, 75% of whom are between the ages of 55 and 84 years. Stroke, which typically refers to an event of blockage of blood supply to a particular part of the brain, represents the 3rd most frequent cause of death in the United States. Approximately 1/3 of stroke victims do not survive the initial attack. Of those who do, only 10% are able to return to work without disability. Another 40% will experience a mild disability, while an additional 40% are severely disabled. A full 10% of stroke survivors will spend the rest of their lives institutionalized because of their inability to carry out activities of self-care.[1]

In the United States, medical expenditures for the care of stroke patients exceeds $30 billion annually. But the emotional impact on patients, their families and caregivers is incalculable.[2]

Homocysteine and Stroke Prevention

Over the past 30 years there has been a small but certainly meaningful reduction in stroke incidence in this country. No doubt this is due, to some degree, to an increased awareness of, and attention to, several well-recognized risk factors including high blood pressure, cigarette smoking, diabetes, and elevated cholesterol.

But while attention to the role of these medical conditions in increasing susceptibility to stroke is important, recent medical research has identified an even more profound risk factor. *Homocysteine*, an amino acid generated during the normal course of protein digestion, is now recognized as a critical factor in increasing the risk of stroke as well as coronary artery disease.

Elevation of homocysteine in the blood dramatically increases the production of atheromatous plaque – a mixture of fat and calcified inflammatory tissue that progressively narrows arteries. When the arteries supplying the brain are compromised by this process, the stage is set for the often catastrophic event we know as a stroke.

It is unclear why homocysteine has received so little attention until just the past 5 years. Indeed, its pivotal role in vascular disease was first described over 30 years ago by Dr. Kilmer McCully – research that earned him the 1998 Linus Pauling Award.[3] Following his landmark publication, other researchers soon discovered a direct relationship between increased homocysteine and stroke risk.[4,5]

In a study regarded as providing the most definitive understanding of the relationship between elevation of homocysteine and stroke risk, researchers at *Tufts University* measured blood homocysteine levels and the degree of narrowing of the carotid arteries (one of the main arteries to the brain) in 1,041 elderly men and women. Narrowing of the carotid arteries was measured using ultrasound – a noninvasive technique commonly employed in assessing stroke risk. The results clearly indicated a significantly increased risk of extensive arterial narrowing in the subjects with the highest homocysteine levels as seen in the figure 7.1.[6]

In contrast to elevated cholesterol, hypertension and diabetes, stroke risk factors for which the causes may be obscure, what leads to elevation of homocysteine has now been well defined. Quite simply, homocysteine levels reflect the intake of 3 important vitamins, B6, B12, and, folic acid. Inadequacies of any one or more of these nutrients can enhance homocysteine production, leading to an increased risk of stroke. Perhaps this explains why the role of homocysteine is not yet generally appreciated by mainstream medicine. For unlike problems with blood pressure, diabetes or cholesterol, the remedy for high homocysteine isn't provided via the prescription pad. The fix for the problem requires simple and inexpensive vitamin administration.

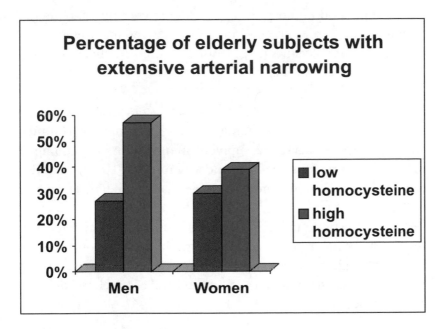

Figure 7.1. Narrowing of the carotid arteries and blood homocysteine levels. From: Selhub, J., et al., N Engl J Med 322(5): 286-291, 1995

It has only been in recent years that the powerful role of vitamin supplementation in terms of disease prevention has appeared in the medical literature. In an important study published in the *Journal of the American Medical Association* in 1993 entitled *"Vitamin Status and Intake as Primary Determinants of Homocysteinemia in an Elderly Population,"* researchers from *Tufts University* revealed how widespread deficiencies of vitamins B6, B12 and folic acid in the elderly produces elevated homocysteine and so increases risk of stroke and other vascular problems. As the authors stated, "… a strong case can be made for prevention of the marginal or manifest vitamin deficiency states that may contribute substantially to this potentially important risk factor for vascular disease, the largest cause of mortality in elderly individuals. Efforts to prevent deficiencies of folate, vitamin B12, and vitamin B6 in the increasing number of our population over the age of 65 years now have added impetus."[1]

Evaluating blood homocysteine is as easy as checking cholesterol. Like the cholesterol test, checking homocysteine requires an overnight fast. Normal values range from 8-14 μmol/L , but a level below 10 should be the goal.

If elevated, homocysteine can almost always be normalized with relatively small amounts of B vitamins. In a recent study of 100 men with elevated homocysteine, supplementation with just 0.65mg of folic acid, 0.4mg vitamin B12, and vitamin B6 (10mg) each day resulted in a reduction of homocysteine by an incredible 50% ! [2]

Because of the profound implications of elevated homocysteine, this test should be incorporated into the general physical examination of every adult. Certainly every stroke patient should be screened for elevated homocysteine as its causal role in stroke is so clearly defined, and its remedy so facile.

Healing with Oxygen

Up until just recently, the commonly accepted teaching with respect to stroke recovery held that because the adult brain lacked *plasticity* (the ability of brain tissue to take over the function of a damaged area), there was essentially no chance of any meaningful functional recovery following a stroke or other brain injury after the first few months. But new scientific research reveals that this pessimistic view is clearly unwarranted.

In a presentation at the 51st Annual Meeting of the American Academy of Neurology, researchers from the *University of Kansas Medical Center* reported that the brain has significant potential for recovery following injury. As Dr. Randolph J. Nudo of the research team stated, " We are now beginning to think that the six-month end point is not final. There may be ways to perturb the system so that further recovery can occur. If in fact we can introduce other therapeutic techniques during some presumed critical period, we may be able to enhance recovery in even the moderate to severe cases." [3]

It is this new understanding of the brain's ability to regain function that supports the therapeutic techniques described in the BrainRecovery.com protocol for stroke recovery.

When an individual experiences a stroke, there is by definition a portion of brain tissue that is permanently destroyed – in essence dead. It is critically important to recognize, however, that there is no clear-cut delineation between the dead tissue and tissue which remains fully functional. There exists between these two areas a population of neurons whose function has been diminished by the stroke event, but which nevertheless remain viable. This area, made up of functional but non-functioning tissue, has been termed the "ischemic penumbra" in the scientific literature. Another term more user friendly is to simply refer to these neurons as "idling." They are like cars parked with their motors running at idle – waiting to be put into gear.

Until recently, no efficacious therapy has been available which could specifically target those idling neurons to restore their metabolic function. But over the past decade, stroke therapy in the United States has been revolutionized. It has now become evident in the medical literature that the technique of hyperbaric oxygen therapy (HBOT) can restore some metabolic activity to damaged neurons. This obviously has profound implications for those disabled by a stroke.

Hyperbaric oxygen therapy is an exciting medical treatment approved by both the FDA and the AMA for the treatment of a wide variety of medical disorders. Many may be familiar with HBOT as it is used for the treatment of "the bends" and other diving related injuries. In recent years the therapeutic scope of HBOT has widened considerably and includes a variety of medical problems like thermal burns,

carbon monoxide poisoning, non-healing skin wounds, diabetic ulcers, and radiation injuries to name a few. But while the utility of
HBOT in treating these and other disorders is well accepted in this
country, its utilization in the treatment of stroke and other brain
injuries remains minimal, despite the fact that it is used as first line
therapy for these and other neurological disorders across Europe and
Asia. Indeed West Germany has long recognized the effectiveness of
this therapy in stroke rehabilitation to the extent that now virtually
all stroke patients in West Germany are eligible to receive a 3-week
intensive course of hyperbaric oxygen therapy.

The therapy acts by enhancing tissue levels of life-giving oxygen.
Normally, oxygen is almost exclusively carried by red blood cells.
When an individual receives HBOT therapy, there is a profound
increase in the amount of oxygen carried in all of the body's fluids
including plasma, lymph, intracellular fluids, and cerebrospinal fluid.
This allows increased oxygen levels even in areas with poor or compromised blood supply as well as in areas of tissue damage.

Increasing tissue oxygen levels produces several important long-term
therapeutic benefits including enhanced growth of new blood
vessels, increased ability of white blood cells to destroy bacteria
and remove toxins, enhanced growth of fibroblasts (cells involved
in wound healing), and most importantly in stroke recovery,
enhanced metabolic activity of previously marginally functioning
cells –including neurons.

Hyperbaric oxygen therapy simply means exposing patients to pure
oxygen under increased atmospheric pressure. Patients receiving hyperbaric oxygen therapy enter a chamber in which they breathe 100%
oxygen delivered under increased pressure. During the treatments,
which typically last one to two hours, patients relax, watch television, or sleep while they are carefully monitored by highly trained
technicians with whom they can communicate easily through an intercom system as seen in figure 7.2.

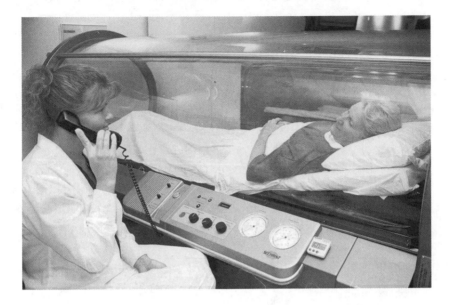

Figure 7.2. The Sechrist model 3200 monoplace chamber is large enough to comfortably accommodate an adult and child.

Since the early 1970's, scientific journalists have reported over 1,000 cases demonstrating a 40% to 100% rate of improvement for stroke patients treated with hyperbaric oxygen therapy. In the highly regarded, peer reviewed journal *Stroke*, Dr. Richard Neubauer, a pioneer in the use of hyperbaric oxygen in various neurological diseases, reported outstanding results in a group of 122 stroke patients treated with hyperbaric oxygen therapy. In one case, significant functional improvement was noted when hyperbaric oxygen therapy was given as late as *14 years* after the initial stroke event.

Typically, the benefits of HBOT for stroke patients include improvements of gait, speech, mental function, motor power, and reduction of spasticity. Dr. Neubauer noted that combining HBOT with physical, occupational and speech therapy where indicated, offered the best chance for improvement.[1] These findings have been confirmed in European studies as seen in table 7.1.

In addition to these measurable parameters, an exciting new technique is now available to graphically demonstrate the effectiveness of hyperbaric oxygen therapy. It involves performing a *functional* scan of the brain known as a SPECT (single photon emission computerized tomography) scan. Unlike familiar CAT scans and MRI scans that simply provide a visual image of anatomy, the SPECT scan is unique in actually identifying and quantifying brain metabolism, both normal and abnormal. SPECT scanning involves the intravenous injection of a radio-labeled chemical. Next, the injection is traced through the brain revealing areas of normal as well as compromised metabolism. This provides an extremely effective way of demonstrating improvements in brain function following the administration of hyperbaric oxygen therapy.

Neurological dysfunction	Number with this dysfunction	Number improved
impaired mental function	35	30 (86%)
gait impairment	24	10 (41%)
motor power impairment	50	50 (100%)
spasticity	21	21 (100%)
speech impairment	8	2 (25%)

Table 7.1. Long Term Results of Treatment of Stroke Patients with Combined HBOT and Physical Therapy[2] From: Jain, K.K., Textbook of Hyperbaric Medicine. Second Edition, Seattle, Hogrefe and Huber, p. 269, 1996

Case Report

Shortly after we began using hyperbaric oxygen therapy we were contacted by a family quite distraught following their father's stroke. The patient, Mr. D., had undergone a coronary bypass operation at a large hospital in Orlando, Florida in May of 1998. Complications ensued toward the end of the procedure with the patient experiencing a cardiac arrest. Following his resuscitation, Mr. D. was completely unresponsive. He then underwent a CAT scan of the brain revealing multiple strokes throughout the brain (see figure 7.3). The patient was then transferred to the intensive care unit on total life support. After several days and no improvement, the attending physician asked if the patient had executed a living will as he had determined that the patient had no chance of any meaningful recovery.

It was at that point that we received a call from the patient's family. They arranged to have me flown to Orlando to assess the situation first hand. As anticipated, based on the nature of the injury, the patient was indeed totally unresponsive and dependent on life support machines. After reviewing the CAT scans and examining the patient, we contacted the attending physician to discuss the possibility of using hyperbaric oxygen therapy as a measure of last resort. Coincidentally, the hospital had a first class hyperbaric oxygen chamber just one floor below.

After overcoming a multitude of bureaucratic roadblocks, the attending physician consented, and Mr. D. was transported to the hyperbaric chamber. Within seconds after beginning the therapy, The patient opened his eyes and began looking around. Upon completion of his first treatment, he was able to follow verbal commands to move his fingers and close his eyes.

He received a total of 14 treatments while in the hospital. Thereafter, the hospital refused further HBOT treatments for reasons that remain unclear.

In early June, Mr. D. was transferred by air ambulance to a nursing home in Naples, Florida so we could continue HBOT at our center. He arrived with a tracheostomy (breathing tube) in his throat, and a feeding tube in his stomach as seen in figure 7.4.

Over the next 6 weeks, in addition to 30 HBOT treatments, Mr.D. received vigorous speech and physical therapy. During that time his tracheostomy and stomach tubes were removed with the patient regaining both the ability to eat solid food and speak (see figure 7.5.).

At the time of transfer to a facility nearer his home, Mr. D. could sit comfortably in a chair and could stand with assistance.

Figure 7.3. Computerized tomographic brain scans of patient E.D. showing multiple infarcts (strokes) of the brain (blue arrows).

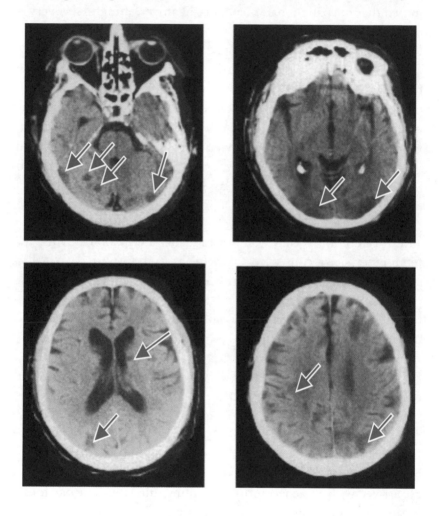

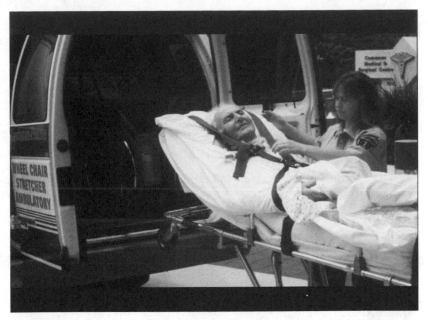

Figure 7.4. Patient E.D. arriving to begin hyperbaric oxygen therapy.

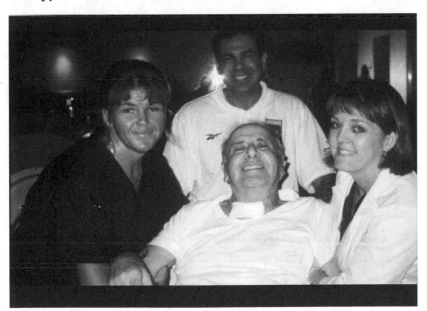

Figure 7.5. Patient E.D. following 30 hyperbaric oxygen treatments.

Cellular Energetics

In contrast to the neurodegenerative conditions described earlier in this text, limiting ongoing free radical injury takes on less importance in a chronic and relatively static brain injury as is seen in stroke. In this type of brain disorder, the main goal is to enhance function of the surviving neurons using specific therapies designed to augment the energy producing activity of the mitochondria and thus enhances their metabolic potential. As noted above, hyperbaric oxygen therapy represents a powerful tool in stroke recovery – acting precisely by this mechanism.

The addition of acetyl-L-carnitine, coenzyme Q10, NADH, phosphatidylserine, and an exciting new discovery, *vinpocetine,* creates a powerful and effective therapeutic program – the **BrainRecovery.com** protocol.

Acetyl-L-carnitine

Brain cell function is directly dependant upon energy availability. Maintaining adequate cellular energy resources requires the efficient delivery of appropriate and sufficient fuel to the mitochondria. By helping to shuttle fuel to the mitochondria, acetyl-L-carnitine plays an essential role in the process of cellular metabolism. In addition to transporting fuel sources into the mitochondria for consumption, acetyl-L-carnitine assists in removing the toxic by-products of cellular metabolism. Because of these functions, acetyl-L-carnitine has a pivotal role in facilitating the fundamental processes necessary for maintaining and enhancing brain cell function.

Coenzyme Q10 (CoQ10), and Nicotinamide Adenine Dinucleotide (NADH)

As noted above, in the brains of stroke patients there exists a population of brain cells surrounding the most severely damaged neurons. These have been called *idling neurons*, a term connoting viability but with compromised function. At the heart of the metabolic infirmity of these neurons is an inadequacy of cellular energy production resulting from damage to the mitochondria – the cellular power plant.

Both CoQ10 and NADH are fundamental requirements in the process of mitochondrial energy production. Increasing the availability of these critical cofactors creates an environment where mitochondrial function is enhanced. This increases energy availability for compromised neurons. The ability of NADH to revitalize the metabolism of damaged neurons likely explains its effectiveness in other neurological conditions including Alzheimer's disease and Parkinson's disease. [1,2]

Animal studies provide compelling insight into the power of coenzyme Q10 in stroke. Experimental occlusion of the carotid artery in the rabbit very rapidly produces multiple areas of brain destruction (stroke) in addition to severe neurological deficits. But if their diets are enriched with CoQ10 prior to occluding the artery, no neurological deficit appears and microscopic evaluation of their brains reveals essentially no evidence of injury. [3]

In this context, it seems reasonable to reevaluate the vigorous approach taken by medical practitioners to lower cholesterol in an attempt to reduce stroke risk since many of the most popular cholesterol lowering drugs not only reduce cholesterol, but deplete coenzyme Q10 levels as well. [4]

Phosphatidylserine

The actual machinery within the mitochondria where fuel is transformed into energy is a fat laden structure - the *mitochondrial membrane*. Phosphatidylserine makes up one of the key components of this structure, thus explaining its pivotal role in neuronal metabolism.

Another important membrane in nervous system tissue surrounds the neuron itself and as such is known as the *neuronal membrane*. As in the mitochondrial membrane, phosphatidylserine is a key building block in the neuronal membrane. Maintaining functional integrity of the neuronal membrane is critical for brain function since this is the site where brain cells both receive and transmit chemical messages.

Phosphatidylserine thus functions both in cellular energy production and at the level of cell-to-cell communication. These vital functions support its inclusion in the **BrainRecovery.com** protocol for stroke recovery.

Vinpocetine

One of the most exciting discoveries in the treatment of stroke patients is vinpocetine, an extract of the lesser periwinkle plant *Vinca minor*. Presently in use in over 35 countries around the world, vinpocetine has been clinically proven to meaningfully improve the clinical outcome of stroke patients, even when administered long after the initial stroke event. In a 1985 Japanese study, researchers demonstrated "slight-to-moderate" improvement in two-thirds of stroke patients receiving this remarkable natural substance.[5]

Vinpocetine's effectiveness in stroke recovery is likely due in part to its remarkable ability to dilate brain arteries, enhancing brain blood flow in patients with cerebrovascular disease.[6] This improves delivery of life-giving oxygen to marginally functioning areas of the brain.

In addition, two other therapeutic qualities of vinpocetine support its inclusion in the **BrainRecovery.com** protocol for stroke recovery. First, vinpocetine acts as a potent antioxidant and thus limits ongoing brain damage from free radical production.[7] Second, vinpocetine reduces the tendency of red blood cells and platelets to aggregate or stick together. This function, coupled with its ability to increase the flexibility of red blood cells, further enhances blood flow to damaged brain areas while reducing the risk of subsequent stroke.[8,9]

BrainRecovery.com
Stroke Recovery Protocol

Homocysteine

As devastating as a stroke may be, the event itself may have one saving grace. It alerts both patient and physician as to the presence of an underlying abnormality of brain blood supply, prompting a review of risk factors. Defining and treating the well recognized risk factors of diabetes, high cholesterol, cigarette smoking, and high blood pressure should not prove challenging to most physicians.

Despite extensive research with frequent medical publications describing the important role of homocysteine in stroke risk, many contemporary physicians remain unaware that a simple blood test for this chemical can not only identify high-risk patients, but may explain why the event occurred. Insist on having a blood test for homocysteine. Elevated homocysteine requires increased amounts of folic acid, and vitamins B6 and B12 (see below). Homocysteine can be evaluated by having your doctor or lab send a blood sample to:

Great Smokies Diagnostic Laboratory
63 Zillicoa Street
Asheville, N.C. 28801-9801
Tel. (800) 522 – 4762

Hyperbaric Oxygen Therapy

HBOT is used worldwide as a powerful adjunct in stroke recovery. More information about its usefulness in stroke and other neurological conditions can be found in chapter nine, and at www.BrainRecovery.com.

Cellular energizers

	daily dose
Coenzyme Q10	150-200mg
Phosphatidylserine	100mg
NADH	5mg (twice)
Acetyl-L-carnitine	400mg
Vinpocetine	5mg (twice)

Vitamins

	daily dose
Folic acid	800 mcg
Vitamin B3	100 mg
Vitamin B6	100 mg
Vitamin B12	200 mcg

Or, if using the Brain Sustain™ supplement:

NADH and Vinpocetine as above, and:

Brain Sustain™ — 2 scoops daily

Coenzyme Q10 — 100mg

Vitamin B12 — 1000mcg
(if homocysteine elevated)

BrainSustain is a nutritional supplement designed to maintain healthy brain function. It is not intended to treat or cure any specific disease.

References

[1] Birkmayer, J.G.D., Coenzyme Nicotinamide Adenine Dinucleotide – New Therapeutic Approach for Improving Dementia of the Alzheimer Type. Ann Clin and Lab Science 26(1):1-9, 1996

[2] Birkmayer, J.G. D., et al, Nicotinamide Adenine Dinucleotide (NADH) – A New Therapeutic Approach to Parkinson's Disease: Comparison of Oral and Parenteral Application. Acta Neurol Scand 87 (146): 32-35 1993

[3] Greib, P., Ryba, M.S., Sawicki, J., et al., Oral coenzyme Q10 administration prevents the development of ischemic brain lesions in a rabbit model of symptomatic vasospasm. Acta Neuropathol (Berl), 4: 363-8, 1997

[4] Mortensen, S.A., Leth, A., Agner, E., Dose-related decrease of serum coenzyme Q10 during treatment with HMG-CoA reductase inhibitors. Mol Aspects of Med 18(Suppl.) S137-44, 1997

[5] Otomo, E., Atarashi, J., Araki, G., et al., Comparison of Vinpocetine with ifenprodil tartrate and dihydroergotoxine mesylate treatment and results of long-term treatment with Vinpocetine. Curr Therapeut Res, 37: 811-821, 1985

[6] Tamaki, N., Kusunoki, T., Matsumoto, S., The effect of Vinpocetine on cerebral blood flow in patients with cerebrovascular disease. Ther Hung , 33: 13-21. 1985

[7] Olah, V.A. Balla, G., Balla, J., et al., An in vitro study of the hydroxyl scavenger effect of caviton. Acta Paediatr Hung, 30: 309-316, 1990

[8] Osawa, M., Maruyama, S., Effects of TCV-3B (Vinpocetine) on blood viscosity in ischemic cerebrovascular disease. Ther Hung, 33: 7-12, 1985

[9] Hayakawa, M., Comparative efficacy of Vinpocetine, pentoxifylline and nicergoline on red blood cell deformability. Arzneimittelforschung, 42: 108-110,1992

CHAPTER EIGHT

Brain Protection and Performance Enhancement

BrainRecovery.com has thus far focused on therapeutic approaches to various neurodegenerative conditions. But clearly, the fundamental concepts of both protecting the brain against the damaging effects of free radicals as well as enhancing the energy producing efficiency of brain neurons have important implications in the preservation and enhancement of brain function in individuals not specifically challenged by a brain disorder.

The brain is uniquely at increased risk for free radical induced damage for several reasons. First, the human brain contains more than 60% fat, a substance known to be highly sensitive to free radicals. In addition, while the brain makes up only about 5% of the adult body weight, it nevertheless consumes an incredible 20% of the oxygen used by the body. This high degree of oxygen utilization markedly increases free radical production. Finally, the brain contains relatively low levels of important antioxidants rendering this most critical organ even more at risk for the damaging effects of free radicals.

The pivotal role of free radicals in aging and degeneration is now generally accepted in the worldwide scientific community.[1] Likewise, the fundamental role of mitochondrial energy failure is now recognized as the key functional impairment responsible for the deficiencies of brain function in virtually all of the important degenerative brain disorders including Alzheimer's disease and Parkinson's disease as described in a recent article appearing in *Scientific American*.[2]

Preserving and enhancing brain function therefore requires appropriate antioxidant protection, along with the provision of the necessary substrates for adequate neuronal energy production. It is interesting to note that many of nutrients described below actually accomplish both tasks. This is understandable since excessive free radical production has a direct detremental effect on the fragile mitochondria, rendering them less able to carry out their critical task of energy production.

Vitamin E

Of the various types of chemicals found within the body, fat is the most susceptible to being damaged by free radicals. This explains why the brain, having such a high content of fat, is at such an increased risk for free radical damage. Vitamin E is a "fat soluble" antioxidant meaning that its protective effect is most realized in tissues with a high fat content - like the brain. This explains why vitamin E has been so extensively studied in such brain disorders as Parkinson's disease and Alzheimer's disease. It is vitamin E's profound ability to limit the damaging action of free radicals in the brain that likely explains why it outperformed a so called "Alzheimer's drug" in a clinical trial of Alzheimer's patients in a 1997 report in the *New England Journal of Medicine*.[3] Indeed, diets rich in natural sources of vitamin E are associated with a reduction in the risk of Parkinson's disease by an incredible 61%.[4] In individuals already given the diagnosis, the progression of Parkinson's disease has been dramatically slowed with vitamin E and C supplementation.[5] Further, in research appearing in the March 2000 issue of *Neurology*, vitamin E supplementation (along with vitamin C) was directly related to preservation of cognitive function as demonstrated in an extensive long-term study involving over 3,000 men. As the authors concluded, " In the current study there was a strong interaction between vitamin E and C in promoting cognitive performance. Previous studies have suggested that a combination of vitamin E and C might provide more antioxidant protection than either alone. It has been suggestes that vitamin C increases vitamin E levels."[6] Always read vitamin E labels carefully and choose *d-alpha tocoherol* as opposed to *dl-alpha tocopherol* as the biological activity of the former greatly exceeds that of the latter.

Gingko biloba

Ginkgo biloba, extracted from the dried green leaves of the Maidenhair tree, has played an integral role in Chinese medicine for more than 5,000 years, and with good reason. Like vitamin E, Gingko biloba, has potent antioxidant activity. It also directly improves brain metabolism and increases brain blood flow. Gingko biloba is clearly one of the most extensively studied nutritional supplements, especially in neurodegenerative conditions. In a placebo-controlled, double-blind randomized trial recently published in the *Journal of the American Medical Association*, not only did Gingko biloba stabilize Alzheimer's disease, but in many of the subjects there was an actual improvement noted in various standardized psychological tests[7]. Its effeciveness was also confirmed in a 6 month double-blind, placebo-controlled trial of 31 middle-aged participants experiencing mild to moderate memory loss. Ginkgo biloba provided a beneficial effect on cognitive function as demonstrated on several tests of neuropsychological function.[8]

It is certainly humbling that while it is doubtful that the ancient Chinese had an understanding of the role of free radicals in brain disorders, they nevertheless were able to recognize the potential of this powerful herb.

Coenzyme Q-10

Coenzyme Q-10 plays an important role in the production of cellular energy and is found in every living cell of every living being. In addition, it serves an important role as a brain antioxidant. In a recent report in the journal *Lancet*, coenzyme Q10 (along with supplemental iron and pyridoxine) was tested in patients with a severe inherited form of dementia and was found to dramatically reverse the deficit. When the supplement program was discontinued, symptoms returned which again abated when the supplement was resumed. In describing one of the patients in the study, the authors stated, "Her daily activity improved from stage 5 (moderate Alzheimer's Disease) to 1 (normal), she had increased blood flow to the cerebral cortex and decreased symptoms of clinical dementia... She now rides a motorcycle."[9]

When administered orally, coenzyme Q10 is readily absorbed and measurably increases the efficiency of cellular energy production as demonstrated in studies performed at the *Massachusetts General Hospital.*[10] This explains why coenzyme Q-10 is being vigorously evaluated at major institutions around the world as a therapeutic aid in brain disorders. Interestingly, Parkinson's disease patients

demonstrate dramatically lowered levels coenzyme Q-10 which may in part explain why these patients experience higher levels of brain damaging free radical activity. [11]

Alpha Lipoic Acid

This exciting antioxidant is the subject of intensive worldwide study in neurodegenerative diseases because of its powerful antioxidant activity as well as its ability to regenerate other important brain antioxidants including vitamins E, C, and glutathione. Unlike other antioxidants, alpha lipoic acid is both fat-soluble and water-soluble. This greatly enhances its ability to be absorbed from the gut and permits increased penetration into the brain where it serves to protect delicate neuronal cellular membranes against free radical damage.[12] Lipoic acid has been studied extensively and demonstrates profound effectiveness in improving survival and reducing the extent of free radical mediated brain injury in laboratory animal stroke models.[13]

N-Acetyl-Cysteine (NAC)

While glutathione represents one of the most important of the brain's antioxidant's defenses, it is generally considered useless when given orally. NAC is readily absorbed from the gut and dramatically increases the body's production of brain protecting glutathione. The ability of NAC to increase brain glutathione is enhanced in the presence of adequate amounts of vitamin C and E. In addition to enhancing glutathione production, NAC itself is a potent antioxidant and has been demonstrated to reduce the formation of the free radical *nitric oxide* which has been implicated as having a causative role in Parkinson's disease, Alzheimer's disease, and several other neurodegenerative disorders. [14]

NAC itself is a potent antioxidant and has been demonstrated to reduce the formation of the free radical nitric oxide

Acetyl-L-Carnitine

Acetyl-L-carnitine is an important component of the BrainRecovery.com **Brain Protection and Performance Enhancement Protocol** because of its important role in facilitating neuronal energy production. This critical nutrient enhances the ability of brain cells to produce energy by functioning as a shuttle - transporting fuel sources into the mitochondria, the energy producing machinery of the neuron. It also assists in removing toxic byproducts of brain metabolism and acts as a potent antioxidant as well.

Various studies have demonstrated that deficiencies of neuronal energy production render brain cells much more susceptible to damage from extrinsic toxins.[15] This explains why acetyl-L-carnitine has been so vigorously studied as a way of protecting the brain against toxic insults and has now been demonstrated to protect laboratory animals from developing parkinsonism when they are exposed to specific chemicals know to induce the disease.[16] It has been extensively studied in Alzheimer's disease and, as reported in a recent issue of the journal *Neurology,* acetyl-L-carnitine can profoundly reduce the rate of progression of Alzheimer's disease in younger patients.[17]

Phosphatidylserine

Research carried out at *Stanford University* evaluating 149 patients suffering from dementia demonstrated that orally administered phosphatidylserine produced a marked improvement on performance tests related to memory and learning.[18] Like acetyl-L-carnitine and coenzyme Q-10, phosphatidylserine plays an important role in maintaining the ability of brain neurons to produce energy. Phosphatidylserine is a fundamental constituent of the fatty membranes surrounding the mitochondria where energy production occurs. In addition, it also serves as a critical component of the membrane surrounding neurons and thus plays a fundamental role in the process by which brain cells both receive and transmit chemical messages thus substantiating the inclusion of phosphatidylserine in any program designed to enhance brain function.

Vitamin D

Deficiencies of vitamin D have been found in Parkinson's disease, multiple sclerosis, and Alzheimer's disease. It is only in the past several years that vitamin D has been recognized as having far more important role in human health than simply aiding bone formation. Vitamin D is now recognized as a potent fat-soluble antioxidant. Several studies have indicated that vitamin D's ability to quench free radicals is even more powerful than vitamin E.[19]

Vitamin B12 (Methylcobalamin)

Deficiency of vitamin B12 has been associated with mental slowness, confusion, depression, memory difficulties, abnormalities of nerve function, Alzheimer's disease, and multiple sclerosis. Not only is vitamin B12 critical for the maintenance of myelin, the protective insulating coat surrounding each neuron, but it also helps reduce the level of a particular amino acid, *homocysteine*, which has been associated with increased risk for Alzheimer's disease, stroke, and myocardial infarction.

Magnesium

This important mineral is critical in a program designed to preserve and enhance brain function for several important reasons. First, adequate amounts of magnesium are necessary for the electrical depolarization of the neuronal membrane. This is the process by which chemical messages are transmitted from one neuron to another. Next, magnesium enhances the function of various brain antioxidants thus helping to protect the brain against free radical damage. Finally, magnesium helps to prevent the production of specific chemicals within the body which increase inflammation. In Alzheimer's disease, Parkinson's disease, and multiple sclerosis, inflammation represents a fundamental mechanism enhancing the formation of brain damaging free radicals.

Folic Acid

A large number of studies have confirmed a direct relationship between folic acid status and various neurological problems including dementia, memory loss, and even depression. Like vitamin B12, the importance of folic acid in preserving normal brain function likely stems from its role in reducing homocysteine. Homocysteine is a toxic amino acid, elevation of which is associated with more rapid deterioration in some forms of dementia as well as a dramatic increase in stroke risk

Pyridoxine

Pyridoxine (vitamin B6) is critical for maintenance of adequate cellular metabolism. Its role in preserving brain function has been demonstrated in several studies showing a direct relationship between low levels of pyridoxine and severity of dementia.[20] Like folic acid and vitamin B12, pyridoxine helps reduce homocysteine.

Niacin (as niacinamide)

Like pyridoxine, niacin (vitamin B3) is a key cofactor in the fundamental process of brain cell energy production. Deficiencies of niacin can profoundly affect brain cell metabolism resulting in dementia.

Vitamin C

Vitamin C represents one of the most important water soluble free radical scavengers in the human body. In addition, it facilitates the recycling of vitamin E, allowing this important fat soluble antioxidant to continue providing important protection to delicate neuronal membranes. The beneficial interplay between these two vitamins was eloquently described in an article entitled, *Association of Vitamin E and C Supplement Use with Cognitive Function in Elderly Men,* appearing in a recent issue of the journal *Neurology* and is summarized above in the discussion of vitamin E.

This important relationship between vitamins C and E serves as an example of a fundamental concept in neuroprotection. All of the important antioxidants and cellular energizers are mutually dependant. No one or few specific nutrients can provide sufficient protection. With exclusion of one of the major components a weak link in the chain is created rendering the brain at increased for free radical mediated damage.

Essential Fatty Acids (EFAs)

As has been repeatedly described throughout this text, the role of essential fatty acids in brain health cannot be overstated. The EFAs serve as basic structural building blocks of neurons, are used as fuel substrates for brain metaboloism, and provide the raw material for the manufacturing of prostaglandins - the fundamental chemical regulators of brain inflammation.

These fats are termed *essential* as they are not manufactured within the human body and are therefore only made available by dietary sources. Diets rich in unrefined grains, dark green leafy vegetables, cold water fish, eggs, and seeds generally provide adequate quantities of these oils. Unfortunately, the modern Western diet is profoundly deficient in sources of essential fatty acids, providing in their place highly modified fats which serve to displace EFAs in both their structural and functional roles.

Essential fatty acids from both the omega 3 and omega 6 groups are therefore mandatory components of this program.

BrainRecovery.com
Brain Protection and Performance Enhancement Protocol

Vitamins, Minerals and Cellular Energizers   <u>daily dose</u>

Vitamin E acetate (d-alpha-tocopherol) _____ 200 IU
Alpha lipoic acid _____ 40 mg
N-acetyl-cysteine _____200 mg
Ginkgo biloba_____30 mg
Phosphatidylserine_____50 mg
Vitamin D_____200 IU
Coenzyme Q-10_____30 mg
Cyanocobalamin (vitamin B12)_____100 mcg
N-acetyl-L-carnitine_____200 mg
Magnesium as citrate_____200 mg
Niacinamide (vitamin B3)_____50 mg
Pyridoxine (vitamin B6)_____50 mg
Vitamin C as ascorbic acid_____400 mg
Folic acid_____400mcg

Essential Fatty Acids   <u>daily dose</u>

Linolenic acid (Omega 3)
    EPA / DHA fish oil providing _____DHA 500 mg
    (see note below)
    and

Linoleic acid   (Omega 6)
    Evening primrose oil, or Borage oil,or
    Black Current oil providing_____GLA 300 mg

> **Or, if using the Brain Sustain™ supplement:**
> Essential fatty acids as above, and:
> **Brain Sustain™**_____1 scoop daily

Two scoops (40 gms) of Brain Sustain™ provide the following:

Vitamin E (d-alpha-tocopherol)_____400 IU
Alpha lipoic acid_____80 mg
N-Acetyl-cysteine_____ 400 mg
Ginkgo biloba extract (leaf) 24% Ginkgo Heterosides____60 mg
Phosphatidylserine_____100 mg
Vitamin D _____ 400 IU
Coenzyme Q-10 _____60 mg
Vitamin B12 (as Methylcobalamin)_____200 mcg
Acetyl-L-carnitine _____400 mg
Magnesium_____20 mg
Vitamin B3 (as Niacin)_____100 mg
Vitamin B6 (as Pyridoxine 5'-Phosphate)_____100 mg
Vitamin C (as Calcium Ascorbate) _____400 mg
Folate (as Folic acid) _____800 mcg
Sodium_____25 mg
Potassium_____20 mg
Calcium_____110 mg
Phosphorus_____190 mg

Other ingredients: Rice protein, rice syrup solids, pure cane molasses, SlimSweet® (lo Han fruit extract), natural flavors, potassium bicarbonate, citric acid, sucralose, SlimSweet® is a registered trademark of TriMedica International, Inc. Does Not Contain: wheat, soy, or corn.

BrainSustain is a nutritional supplement designed to maintain healthy brain function. It is not intended to treat or cure any specific disease.

Note:

The highest quality DHA containing fish oil supplements are manufactured by **Nordic Naturals, Inc.,** and are available by calling *i* **Nutritionals** at: 1-800-530-1982 or by visiting the website www.BrainRecovery.com

These statements have not been evaluated by the Food and Drug Administration. This product is not intended to diagnose, treat, cure or prevent any disease.

References

[1] Harman, D., The Aging Process. Chapter 5 in: Huemer, R.P. ed. The Roots of Molecular Medicine. New York, W.H. Freeman, 75-87; 1986

[2] Wallace, D.C., Mitochondrial DNA in aging and disease. Scient Amer 227: 40-47; 1997

[3] Sano, M., Ernesto, C., Thomas, R.G., et al., A controlled trial of selegeline, alpha-tocopherol, or both as treatment for Alzheimer's disease. N Engl J Med 336:1216-22, 1997

[4] Golbe, L.I., Farrell, T.M., David, P.H., Case-control study of early life dietary factors in Parkinson's disease. Arch Neurol 45(12): 1350-3, 1988

[5] Fahn, S., The endogenous toxin theory of the etiology of Parkinson's disease and a pilot trial of high-dose antioxidants in an attempt to slow the progression of the illness. Ann N Y Acad Sci 570:186-96, 1989

[6] Masaki, K.H., et al., Association of vitamin E and C supplement use with cognitive function and dementia in elderly men. Neurology 54:1265-1272; 2000

[7] Le Bars, P., Katz, M.M., Berman, N., et al., A Placebo-Controlled, Double-blind Randomized Trial of an Extract of Ginkgo Biloba for Dementia. JAMA 278(16):1327-32,1997

[8] Rai, G.S.., et al, A Double-Blind, Placebo-Controlled Study of Ginkgo Biloba Extract (Tanakan) in Elderly Outpatients With Mild to Moderate Memory Impairment. Current Medical Research and Opinion, 12(6):350-355; 1991

[9] Imagawa, M., et al., Coenzyme Q10, Iron and Vitamin B6 in Genetically- Confirmed Alzheimer's Disease.The Lancet 340:671; September 12, 1992

[10] Schults, C.W., Beal, M.F., Fontaine, K. et al., Absorption, tolerability and effects on mitochondrial activity of oral coenzyme Q10 in parkinsonian patients, Neurology 50: 793-795,1998

[11] Schults, C.W., Haas, R.H., Passov, D., Beal, M.F., Coenzyme Q10 Levels Correlate with the Activities of Complexes I and II/III in Mitochondria from Parkinsonian and Nonparkinsonian Subjects. Ann Neurol 42:261-264,1997

[12] Marangon, K., Devaraj, S., Tirosh, O., et al., Comparison of the effect of a-lipoic acid and a-tocopherol supplementation on measures of oxidative stress. Free Radical Biology & Medicine 27(9/10): 1114-1121, 1999

[13] Panigrahi, M., et al., Alpha -Lipoic Acid Protects Against Reperfusion Injury Following Cerebral Ischemia in Rats. Brain Research 717:184-188; 1996

[14] Pahan, K., Sheikh, G.S., Nmboodiri, A.M.S., et al., N-acetyl cysteine inhibits induction of NO production by endotoxin or cytokine stimulated rat peritoneal macrophages, C6 glial cells and astrocytes. Free Radical Biology and Medicine 24(1):39-48, 1998

[15] Swerdlow, R., Origin and functional consequences of the complex I defect in Parkinson's disease. Annals of Neurology   40: 663-671;1996

[16] Steffen, V., Santiago, M., de la Cruz, C.P., et al, Effect of intraventricular injection of 1-methyl-4-phenylpyridinium protection by acetyl-L-carnitine. Human Exp Toxicol 14:865-871,1995

[17] Thal, L.J., Carta, A., Clarke, W.R., et al., A 1-year multicener placebo-controlled study of acetyl-L-carnitine in patients with Alzheimer's disease. Neurology 47:705-711, 19965(Suppl. 1): 65-70, 1993

[18] Crook, T.H., Tinklenberg, J., Yesavage, J., Effects of phosphatidylserine in age-associated memory impairment. Neurology 41:644-49, 1991

[19] Sardar, S., Chakraborty, A., and Chatterjee, M., Comparative effectiveness of vitamin D3 and dietary vitamin E on peroxidation of lipids and enzymes of the hepatic antioxidant system in Sprague - Dawley rats. Int J Vitam Nutr Res, 66(1): 39-45, 1996

[20] Haller, J., Vitamins for the Elderly: Reducing Disability and Improving Quality of Life. Aging Clinical and Experimental Research,

CHAPTER NINE

Hyperbaric Oxygen Therapy

The use of hyperbaric oxygen therapy (HBOT) in the treatment of select neurological disorders is providing tens of thousands of patients a powerful technique to facilitate the healing process. While seemingly new on the scene, the roots of hyperbaric medicine go back centuries.

In 1662 a British clergyman constructed what was likely the first hyperbaric device designed to expose patients to increased atmospheric pressure for therapeutic purposes. The 1800's saw a proliferation of hyperbaric devices across Europe with various therapeutic claims being made without any specific scientific validation.

In 1879 Fontaine, a French surgeon, built a hyperbaric chamber mounted on wheels which served as a mobile operating room. His work demonstrating improved success with hernia repair provided the first data able to stand the test of scientific scrutiny. [1]

It was not until the 1950's that a major addition to the field of hyperbaric medicine dramatically enhanced its therapeutic potential. Up until then, virtually all hyperbaric chambers were simply pressurized with air. But in 1956 researchers in Amsterdam published their results of various surgical procedures carried out in a hyperbaric chamber with one simple but profound modification – oxygen was added. It was the addition of oxygen to the pressurized environment of the hyperbaric chamber that dramatically enhanced the healing properties of this modality and paved the way for the ever increasing scope of illnesses effectively treated with this therapy that we see today.

While HBOT has become a widely accepted form of therapy in such diverse conditions as carbon monoxide poisoning, poorly healing wounds, burn therapy, and diving injuries, its application to neurological diseases is a relatively recent development. But understanding the biological activity of HBOT in the nervous system has provided the rational for exploring the utility of this FDA and AMA approved therapy in a variety of neurological conditions (see table 9.1).

Table 9.1. Rationale for use of HBOT in Neurological Disorders

- **Reduction of hypoxia (oxygen deficiency)**
- **Improvement of microcirculation**
- **Preservation of partially damaged tissue**
- **Improvement of brain metabolism**

From: Jain, K.K., Textbook of Hyperbaric Medicine. Second Edition, Seattle, Hogrefe and Huber, p. 241, 1996

The profound effectiveness of HBOT in the treatment of multiple sclerosis and stroke is well documented in the medical literature as described in chapters two and seven respectively. In addition to these problems, HBOT is proving valuable in the treatment of many other challenging brain disorders as described below.

Cerebral Palsy

The term "cerebral palsy" is not a specific diagnosis, but is now generally applied to children who experience some form of brain trauma either at the time of birth or shortly before. Most commonly these children manifest some degree of cognitive dysfunction along with physical impairment, often weakness and spasticity of arms and legs.

Treatment approaches for children with cerebral palsy (C.P.) are generally directed at the manifestations of the underlying brain disorder. That is, most efforts are geared to increasing range of motion, reducing spasticity, and increasing strength, along with specific therapies designed to enhance skills of communication and academic performance.

As in stroke and head injury, the damaged areas of the brain in cerebral palsy do not exist in sharp contrast to regions of completely normal function. Rather, between these two extremes there exists a population of neurons that while alive, are not functioning at optimum capacity. It is these "idling neurons" that respond to HBOT.

The damaged areas of the brain in cerebral palsy do not exist in sharp contrast to regions of completely normal function.

Evidence accumulating from around the globe is now providing strong support for the use of hyperbaric oxygen therapy (HBOT) as an approach to the actual functional problem in children with cerebral palsy – a technique that targets marginally functioning brain tissue.

Encouraging research is taking place in Canada where Dr. Pierre Marois and his team of researchers at McGill University in Montreal have recently studied 25 children with cerebral palsy, aged 4 to 7 years, treated with hyperbaric oxygen therapy on a daily basis for 20 days. Another 15 children were treated twice a day for 10 days. Both groups thus received a total of 20 treatment sessions. The results of their post-treatment evaluations were truly remarkable. According to Dr. Marois: "…the results are really incredible! Twenty-three of the 25 children have great results. Twenty-three have amelioration with their spasticity and may have amelioration with speech and cognitive function." Further, their published results reveal "the clinical observations do list numerous functional changes, definite improvements, a large amount in the level of arousal/response to communication. From statistical analysis of the objective estimations we confirm these change, more particularly on the level of motor functioning like walking and the quality of sitting position, similarly on the level of spasticity. These results are surprising considering the small number of treatments (20), and of extreme importance because it's the first study documenting objectively the prospects of beneficial effects of HBO in the treatment of children suffering from cerebral palsy." [2] While it is important to recognize that hyperbaric oxygen therapy clearly represents an important tool in the treatment of children with cerebral palsy, it should be viewed as an adjunctive form of therapy to be used in conjunction with other established treatment protocols including physical therapy, occupational therapy, speech therapy, as well as pharmaceutical therapy designed to reduce spasticity. The use of HBO in children with cerebral palsy is now gaining a strong foothold in the United States and there is no doubt that because of its profound effects, its utilization will become much more widespread.

Public awareness of the use of hyperbaric oxygen therapy in children with cerebral palsy in North America can be credited in large part to the work done by Mothers United for Moral Support (MUMS). This worldwide organization, founded by Julie Gordon, a mother of a child with cerebral palsy, seeks to unite parents of children with cerebral palsy and other needs and to share information concerning various therapeutic options.

They can by contacted by telephone at 920-336-5333. E-Mail can be directed to the MUMS National Parent – 2 – Parent network by contacting MUMs@netnet.net.

Closed Head Injury

In an article entitled "Hyperbaric Oxygen for Treatment of Closed Head Injury" appearing in the *Southern Medical Journal*, pioneering researcher Dr. Richard Neubauer revealed the profound potential of HBOT in the treatment of these often catastrophic injuries. As he stated, "Brain injuries, regardless of their cause, share common pathophysiologic pathways that result in the destruction of neurons, and, to varying extent, formation of 'idling neurons.' " [3]

Thus, the rationale for the use of HBOT in head injured patients is much like that described for the treatment of stroke in chapter seven. That is, surrounding the area of maximal injury there exists a population of neurons that while alive are not fully functional. These are the so called idling neurons that seem to respond so readily to hyperbaric oxygen therapy. It is the improvement in function of these neurons that likely explains the effectiveness of HBOT as demonstrated in clinical studies. [4]

Here is a report from the mother of a 16 year old boy who sustained a head injury in a roller skating accident. He was rendered unconscious and subsequently experienced significant cognitive problems affecting his school performance. He was treated with hyperbaric oxygen therapy as well as Ginkgo biloba, vitamin B12, acetyl-L-carnitine, and phosphatidylserine:

> Dear Dr. Perlmutter:
>
> I would like to bring you up-to-date on my son's progress since his treatment in December.
>
> He had his annual school evaluation in June which was given by the same teacher using the same testing materials as she has always used. Joshua jumped 4 grade levels in reading so that he maxed out of the test and is at college level in that subject. Since we began schooling in January until his test in June, he jumped 2 grade levels in math. Before, he was going backward, but now he's leaping over grade levels. Thank you! Also, now that we've started back after summer break, Josh has retained his proficiency in math and can go on from there rather than review for 2 months as before. We have noticed a great maturing in him as well, for which we are very grateful. I realize that these results are purely subjective, however, we know our son better than any clinician could ever know him and we see the results.
>
> Again, thank you and God bless you all.
>
> Sincerely,
>
> J.L.

Bell's Palsy

Bell's palsy is a relatively common medical problem which manifests as a fairly sudden onset of weakness of one side of the face. While the actual cause is still unknown, most researchers agree that a virus may be playing a role by causing inflammation and swelling of the nerve supplying the muscles of the face. This renders these muscles weak which disfigures the face – sometimes permanently.

Because inflammation of the facial nerve leads to weakness, the common approach to the treatment of Bell's palsy has involved the use of anti-inflammatory steroid drugs like prednisone. But with the knowledge that HBOT also dramatically reduces inflammation, researchers explored the use of hyperbaric oxygen compared to the standard prednisone therapy. The results, published in 1997, revealed that the risk of permanent facial weakness from Bell's palsy when

The risk of permanent facial weakness from Bell's palsy when treated with prednisone was 24% compared with only 5% in patients receiving HBOT.

treated with prednisone was 24% compared with only 5% in patients receiving HBOT. The average time to complete recovery was 22 days in those getting HBOT, while it was 34 days in the prednisone group.[5] The other obvious advantage of HBOT over prednisone is the lack of side effects frequently associated with steroid administration.

Chronic Lyme Disease

Lyme disease is an infectious disease transmitted by the bite of a tick. Initial symptoms may include a peculiar "bulls-eye" skin rash, malaise, headache, Bell's palsy (see above) and joint pain. Most patients experience a complete remission once the diagnosis is made and the appropriate antibiotic is administered. But a small percentage of patients experience a relapse of symptoms despite repeated courses of antibiotics. It is these unfortunate individuals who receive the diagnosis of chronic Lyme disease.

Symptoms of chronic Lyme disease may be similar to that of the acute illness but more commonly include persistent fatigue, sleep disturbance, cognitive disorder, personality changes and even painful nerve inflammation.[6]

"It seems clear that HBOT improves or eliminates the symptoms in patients who have been on antibiotics for several years."

Until recently, the only therapy available to treat chronic Lyme disease was a virtual continuous course of powerful antibiotics, often given intravenously. But new research has revealed that the organism causing the disease may be sensitive to oxygen. This has provided the groundwork for the evaluation of hyperbaric oxygen therapy as a treatment for chronic Lyme disease.

In studies being carried out at *Texas A & M University*, Drs. William Fife and Donald Freeman have reported significant improvements in patients with chronic Lyme disease receiving HBOT. Concerning their research they have concluded, " It can be said that the HBOT protocol used in this preliminary study reduces the symptoms and greatly improves the quality of life...It seems clear that HBOT improves or eliminates the symptoms in patients who have been on antibiotics for several years and who have shown no further improvement in the disease symptoms with antibiotics. This suggests that the further improvement seen is due to HBOT which is the only thing changed in the longstanding treatment regimen and which is at least a valid adjunctive treatment to antibiotics." [7]

HBOT offers new hope to those suffering from this chronic illness. As these authors described, HBOT may be used in conjunction with antibiotics to provide chronic Lyme patients the best chance of ridding themselves of this debilitating illness.

What's Involved in Hyperbaric Oxygen Treatment

HBOT treatments, generally lasting from 60 – 90 minutes, are most commonly given in a "monoplace" chamber - so named as they are designed to treat one adult at a time. Under the direction of a trained technician and with the supervision of a physician, the entire chamber is slowly pressurized with 100% oxygen until the appropriate level of pressure is attained. During the pressurization phase, patients are asked to swallow or drink water to help clear their ears much as they would do when flying. Ear equalization is easily accomplished in more than 95% of patients. In those few who have difficulty, surgical placement of temporary ear tubes may be required. Ear tubes are especially useful in the very young or in those patients whose neurological status prevents normal communication.

During the treatment, communication is maintained using an intercom system. Patients sleep or may watch a movie and generally report feeling quite comfortable (see photos chapter seven).

Prior to HBOT, most centers require patients to undergo a chest x-ray in addition to a general physical exam. While it is interesting to note that hyperbaric oxygen therapy actually reduces free radical production and enhances the activity of the antioxidant glutathione[8], the antioxidants vitamin E and N-acetyl-cysteine are typically provided prior to treatment. More about hyperbaric oxygen therapy can be found at www.BrainRecovery.com and in chapter seven.

References

[1] In: *Hyperbaric Medicine Practice*. Kindwall, E., (ed.) Flagstaff, Best Publishing, page 2, 1995

[2] Marois, P., The Pilot Project on Treatment in Hyperbaric Oxygen Therapy. The Reflection – Hospital Marie Enfant 11(3), 1999

[3] Neubauer, R.A., Gottlieb, S.F., and Pevsner, N.H. Hyperbaric Oxygen for the Treatment of Closed Head Injury. Southern Medical Journal 87(9): 933-936, 1994

[4] Jain, K.K., in: *Textbook of Hyperbaric Medicine*. Second Edition, Seattle, Hogrefe and Huber, p. 298, 1996

[5] Racic, G., Denoble, P.J., Sprem, N., et al., Hyperbaric oxygen as a therapy of Bell's palsy. Undersea Hyperbab Med 24(1): 35-8, 1997

[6] Bujak DI, Weinstein A, Dornbush RL. Clinical and neurocognitive features of the post Lyme syndrome. J Rheumatol 1996;23:1392-7

[7] Fife, W.P., and Freeman, D.M., Preliminary Clinical Study on the Use of Hyperbaric Oxygen Therapy for the Treatment of Lyme Disease. (in print), Texas A & M University, Revised February, 1997

[8] Baiborodov, B.D., Savel'eva, T.V., Prokopenko, V.M., et al., Effects of hyperbaric oxygenation and antioxidant system of blood in the newborn who had hypoxia at birth

About the Author

David Perlmutter, M.D. received his M.D. degree from the University of Miami School of Medicine where he was awarded the Leonard G. Rowntree Research Award in 1979. After completing residency training Neurology, also at the University of Miami, Dr. Perlmutter entered private practice in Naples, Florida and received Board Certification in Neurology and Psychiatry in 1987.

Dr. Perlmutter has contributed extensively to the world medical literature with publications appearing in such journals as *The Journal of Neurosurgery, The Southern Medical Journal,* and *Archives of Neurology.* He is recognized internationally as a leader in the field of nutritional influences in neurological disorders and has been interviewed on many nationally syndicated radio and television programs including *20/20, The Faith Daniels Program,* and *Larry King Live.*

In addition to serving as Medical Director for *The Perlmutter Health Center, Perlmutter Hyperbaric Centers,* and *Naples MRI,* Dr. Perlmutter is a member of the Adjunct Faculty at the *Institute for Functional Medicine,* in Gig Harbor, Washington. He is an active member of the *American Medical Association,* the *American Academy of Neurology,* the *American Holistic Medical Association,* the *American College for the Advancement of Medicine,* the *Undersea and Hyperbaric Medical Society,* the *Oxygen Society,* the *American College of Nutrition,* the *Physician's Committee for Responsible Medicine,* and serves on the Medical Advisory Board for *The Integrative Medical Consult.*

Dr. Perlmutter, his wife Leize, and children Austin and Reisha live in Naples, Florida where he continues to practice.

Glossary

Acetyl-L-Carnitine. An important component in the process of cellular energy production. acetyl-L-Carnatine functions to provide fatty fuels for mitochondrial energy production and also assists in removing the byproducts of this process.

Alpha Lipoic Acid. A powerful antioxidant having excellent absorption from the gut and brain penetration.

Alzheimer's disease. A neurodegenerative condition characterized by a progressive deterioration of mental function.

Amyotrophic lateral sclerosis. A neurodegenerative disease characterized by progressive loss of motor function.

Antioxidant. Any one of a large group of natural or synthetic substances that combine with damaging free radical molecules and neutralize them. Important antioxidants include vitamins C, D, and E, alpha lipoic acid, and glutathione.

Arachidonic Acid. A type of fat found in animal products associated with increased inflammation.

Blood-Brain Barrier. A protective layer of cells that excludes many chemicals from reaching the brain.

Borage Seed Oil. A natural oil high in Omega 6 fatty acids useful in reducing inflammation.

Candida albicans. A form of yeast associated with autoimmune diseases and multiple sclerosis.

Cerebral Palsy. A syndrome caused by brain damage during development or at the time of birth.

Chlamydia pneumoniae. A bacterium now associated with multiple sclerosis and other autoimmune disorders.

Coenzyme Q-10 (CoQ10). A critical cofactor in the process of energy production. It also serves as an antioxidant.

Creatine. A substrate for cellular metabolism. Supplemental creatine has been found to increase strength in patients with various neurological disorders.

Doxycycline. An antibiotic useful in the treatment of *Chlamydia pneumoniae.*

Eicosapentanoic Acid (EPA). Part of the Omega 3 essential fatty acid group, EPA has significant anti-inflammatory activity.

Evening Primrose Oil. A natural oil high in Omega 6 fatty acids useful in reducing inflammation.

Flax Seen Oil. A natural oil high in Omega 3 essential fatty acids associated with reduction of inflammation.

Folic Acid. An important water-soluble vitamin. Deficiencies of folic acid are associated with developmental abnormalities of the nervous system as well as elevation of homocysteine.

Gamma Linolenic Acid (GLA). A member of the Omega 6 group with potent anti-inflammatory activity.

Gingko biloba. An ancient Chinese herb now recognized to have significant brain antioxidant activity.

Glutathione. An important brain antioxidant and cofactor in liver detoxification processes.

Homocysteine. An amino acid found in the blood directly related to increased risk of stroke, vascular dementia, Alzheimer's disease, and myocardial infarction.

Human Growth Hormone. A substance normally produced in the brain which directly controls the growth of tissue.

Hyperbaric Oxygen Therapy (HBOT). The administration of oxygen under pressure to promote healing.

Idling Neurons. Brain cells that are metabolically active, but functionally inactive.

Lactobacillus acidophilus. A bacterium that normally resides in the gut and plays an important role in maintenance of intestinal health.

Lyme Disease. A tick born illness often associated with arthritis and neurological problems. It is generally treatable with antibiotics, but may become chronic.

Melatonin. A powerful brain antioxidant normally produced in the pineal gland.

Mitochondria. Microscopic particles within cells responsible for utilizing fuel to provide energy for cellular metabolism.

Multiple Sclerosis. A degenerative condition of the nervous system characterized by loss of myelin.

Myelin. The fragile protective insulation covering surrounding brain neurons.

N-Acetyl-Cysteine (NAC). A nutritional supplement which functions as an antioxidant and enhances glutathione production.

Neurodegenerative Diseases. A group of conditions characterized by progressive deterioration of the central nervous system. Common neurodegenerative diseases include Alzheimer's disease, Parkinson's disease, amyotrophic lateral sclerosis, and multiple sclerosis.

Niacinamide. See Vitamin B3

Nicotinamide Adenine Dinucleotide (NADH). An enzyme which has a pivotal role in energy production in all living cells.

Nitric Oxide. A potent brain damaging free radical.

Parkinson's disease. A neurodegenerative condition characterized by a progressive tremor, rigidity, and difficulties with ambulation.

Phosphatidylserine. A key component of neuronal and mitochondrial membranes.

Post-Polio Syndrome. A disease characterized by progressive weakness in individuals previously afflicted with polio.

Prostaglandins. Derivatives of the essential fatty acids which play an important role in controlling the immune system.

Pyridoxine. See Vitamin B6.

Silymarin (milk thistle). An herb useful in enhancing hepatic detoxification. Silymarin increases the retention of glutathione.

Stroke. Brain damaged caused by a localized interruption of blood supply.

Vinpocetine. An extract of the periwinkle plant which increases brain blood flow and brain cell matabolism.

Vitamin B3. A water soluble vitamin having an important role in energy production. (Niacin – Niacinamide)

Vitamin B6. A water soluble vitamin having an important role in cnergy production. (Pyridoxine)

Vitamin B12. A B vitamin important in the maintenance of myelin, the protective coating over neurons. Vitamin B12 helps reduce homocysteine.

Vitamin C. A water soluble antioxidant.

Vitamin E. A fat soluble antioxidant vitamin important for protecting the brain against free radical damage.

Index

A

Acetaminophen 20, 33, 107, 108, 117, 124
Acetyl-L-carnitine 7, 27, 30, 34, 71, 80, 91, 96, 115, 120, 125, 130, 144, 148, 155,159, 160, 169
Acetylcholine 115
Alcohol 49, 59
ALS (See Amyotrophic Lateral Sclerosis)
Aluminum 1, 103–106, 117, 121, 123, 124
Alzheimer's disease 1, 5, 6, 7, 10, 22, 26, 27, 71, 74, 76, 92, 93, 99–117, 123, 124, 125, 127, 130, 145, 151, 152, 153, 154, 155, 156, 159, 162, 163, 175
Alzheimer's drugs 1, 99
Amyotrophic Lateral Sclerosis 5, 67– 78, 80–83
Antioxidant 4–7, 13, 14, 18, 22, 24–28, 30, 34, 35, 51, 52, 60, 62, 70, 72–76, 79, 83, 92–96, 105, 108, 110, 112, 113, 114, 117, 118, 119, 128, 129, 130, 146, 151–155, 156, 162, 168, 169, 171, 172, 173, 175
Arachidonic acid 108, 109, 175
Aricept® 100
Autoimmune disease 45
Avorn, Jerry 47, 66, 101, 123

B

Bactrim® 22, 34, 82, 107, 123, 125
Beal, Flint M. 22, 34, 70, 82, 123, 125
Beta amyloid 102, 123
Birkmayer, Jörg 21, 34, 114, 125, 149
Black current seed oil 48
Borage oil 48, 62, 119
Brain trauma 7, 164
Bromocriptine 19

C

Candida albicans 40, 41, 61, 175
Cellular phones 101
Cerebral palsy 7, 8, 166, 168, 175
Chlamydia pneumoniae 38, 39, 40, 60, 61, 65, 175
Cholesterol 22, 48, 49, 87, 114, 133–136, 145, 147
Coenzyme Q10 7, 22, 23, 27, 30, 34, 55, 60, 63, 70, 71, 80, 82, 91, 96, 98, 113, 114, 120, 125, 130, 144, 148, 149,155, 159, 160, 162, 175
Cognex ® 1, 100
Comprehensive Digestive Stool Analysis 41, 61

Cortisone 45
Creatine 40, 50, 56, 57, 71, 74, 76, 77, 80, 84, 90, 91, 94, 96, 97, 98, 113, 144, 145, 175
Crohn's disease 42
Cytokines 34, 83, 107, 125
Cytoxan® 45

D

Detoxification 5, 18, 19, 20, 31, 33, 61, 73, 80, 81
DHA 48, 49, 60, 62, 110, 119
Diflucan® 61
Donepezil 100
Dopamine 12, 17, 21–23, 27, 114
Doxycycline 40, 60, 61
Dworkin, Robert 47, 66
Dysbiosis Index 41, 42

E

Eldepryl ® 19
Electromagnetic fields 101, 123
Electromagnetic radiation 1, 101–103, 117
EPA 48, 49, 59, 62, 119, 172
Essential fatty acids 45, 47, 50, 52, 53, 57, 59, 62, 63, 108–111, 118–120,158,159
Essential Fatty Acid Panel 63, 110, 120
Evening primrose oil 48, 62, 110, 119, 159, 176

F

Federation of MS Therapy Centres 57
Fluconazole 61
Folic Acid 106, 117, 128, 130, 134–136, 147, 148, 159, 176
Free radicals 3–6, 13, 24, 25, 27, 51, 52, 55, 60, 68, 69, 72, 92–94, 104, 105, 107–113, 117, 118, 123, 125, 151, 154, 156, 158, 172

G

Gehrig, Lou 2, 67
Ginkgo biloba 7, 27, 30, 35, 52, 60, 62, 76, 79, 84, 96, 111, 119, 125, 130, 152, 153, 159, 160, 176
GLA 48, 49, 59, 62, 110, 119, 176
Glutathione 5–7, 12–18, 20, 25, 26, 29, 30, 33, 52, 72, 73, 75, 78, 80–83, 93, 94, 108, 112, 113, 117, 124, 154, 172, 176
Great Smokies Diagnostic Laboratory 20, 31, 41, 61, 63, 73, 80, 110, 120, 131, 147

H

Helicobactor pylori 39
Homocysteine 54, 106, 107, 116, 117, 124, 125, 127, 128, 130–136, 147, 148, 156, 157, 176
Human growth hormone 77, 79, 80, 87–90, 96, 97, 176
Hyperbaric oxygen therapy 8, 55, 58, 59, 61, 66, 137–141, 143, 144, 147, 176

I

Idling neurons 7, 134, 144, 176
Inflammation 5, 7, 39, 40, 42, 46, 48, 49, 59, 60, 87, 102, 107–110, 118, 158, 170, 171, 175, 176
Insulin-like growth factor (IGF-1) 86
Interferon 45, 86
Interferon-beta 39
Iron 5, 25, 67, 75, 88, 112, 123, 125

K

Klatz, Ronald 81, 84, 87, 97, 98
Kurtzke scale 57

L

L-dopa 12–14, 19, 21, 25, 28
Lactobacillus acidophilus 41, 61, 176
Lauer, Klaus 44, 66
Linoleic acid 46–48, 51, 59, 62, 66, 119,159
Linolenic acid 46, 48, 49, 59, 62, 119,159
Lipoic acid 6, 7, 18, 25, 30, 51, 52, 60, 62, 63, 75, 79, 83, 93, 94, 96, 112, 119, 130
Lovastatin 22, 114

M

Magnesium 60, 63, 110, 120, 156,159,160
Marie, Pierre 37, 65
Massachusetts General Hospital 22, 70, 153
McCully, Kilmer 134
MediClear® 19, 31, 81
Melatonin 105, 117, 119, 120, 123, 124, 176
Memory loss 116, 122
Methotrexate 39, 45
Mevacor® 22, 114
Mirapex® 15
Mitochondria 4–7, 23, 28, 34, 55, 69, 71, 82, 91, 115, 116, 123, 125, 144, 145, 174

MPTP, 27, 35

Multiple sclerosis 5, 7, 8, 37–51, 53, 55, 57–59, 61–66, 68, 74, 83, 87, 109, 175, 176

Myelin 5, 45, 50,51, 53, 57, 65, 116, 176

N

N-acetyl-cysteine, (NAC) 7, 18, 26, 30, 34, 52, 62, 79, 83, 94, 96, 112, 119, 125, 130, 154, 159,160, 172, 177

NADH 7, 21, 22, 27, 30, 34, 54, 60, 63, 92, 96, 97, 114, 120, 130, 144, 145, 148, 149, 177

Neubauer, Richard 139, 168, 173

Newman, P.E. 108, 124

Niacin 71, 157, 159, 177

Nitric oxide 26, 74, 113, 177

Nordic Naturals, Inc. 63, 120, 161

P

Parkinson, James 12

Parkinson's disease 2, 5, 11–19, 21–29, 31–35, 52, 68, 74, 83, 92–94, 107, 124, 145, 149, 152, 153, 163, 177

Parlodel® 19

Pauling, Linus 76, 84, 134

Pesticide 5, 19

Phosphatidylserine 7, 21, 23, 24, 30, 34, 54, 55, 60, 63, 71, 80, 82, 115, 116, 120, 125, 130, 144–146, 148, 155, 159, 160, 177

Pravachol® 22, 114

Pravastatin 22, 114

Prednisone 45, 166

Prostaglandins 45, 416, 49, 59, 177

Pryse-Phillips, William 99, 100, 123

R

Reynolds, E.H. 53, 66

Riluzole 69–71, 83

S

Selegiline 19, 110

Septra® 107

Siegel, Dr. Bernie v

Silymarin 18, 31, 81, 177

Sinemet® 12, 15–17, 19, 21, 25, 107

Sonderdank, Godfried 37

SPECT 140

Sriram, Subramaniam 38, 65

Stress hormones 4
Stroke 7, 68, 127, 128, 133–140, 145–147, 149, 177
Stroke Recovery 8, 133, 136–138, 141, 143–147, 149
Substantia nigra 12
Swank, Roy L. 44, 46, 50, 64, 66

T

Tacrine 1, 10, 100
Tasmar® 15
Tetracycline 40
Thorne Research Inc. 31, 81
Toxins 4, 5, 18, 138
Tremor 11, 14–17, 19, 20, 24, 56, 177
Trowbridge, John 40, 65
Tylenol® 107, 118

U

Ulcerative colitis 42

V

Vascular dementia 106, 127–131
Viagra® 26
Vinpocetine 8, 128–130, 132, 144, 146, 148, 149, 177
Vitamin B12 50, 53, 54, 57, 60, 62, 66, 68, 87, 117, 119, 120, 124, 125,
    130, 136, 148, 156, 159, 160, 169, 177
Vitamin B3 62, 79, 119, 130, 148, 157, 159, 160, 177
Vitamin B6 62, 79, 119, 130, 136, 148, 157, 159, 160, 177
Vitamin C 13, 26, 28, 30, 49, 52, 60, 62, 75, 76, 79, 80, 84, 94, 96, 119,
    130, 152, 154, 157, 160, 162, 177
Vitamin D 27, 30, 34, 51, 52, 60, 62, 66, 74, 75, 79, 83, 95, 98, 113, 119,
    125, 130, 156, 159, 160, 162
Vitamin E 6, 13, 24, 26–28, 30, 35, 52, 59, 60, 62, 69, 70, 74, 75, 79, 80,
    83, 93–97, 110, 111, 113, 119, 130, 152, 154, 156, 157, 158, 159,
    160, 163, 177

W

Weiner, Michael A. 105, 124
Wellness Health and Pharmaceuticals 29, 78, 96

Y

Yeast 40, 41, 43, 65, 171

Z

Zinc 49, 60, 63, 75, 110, 120